EAT FAT, GET FIT

EAT FAT, GET FIT

*How to Create YOUR Perfect Diet
to Lose Weight, Heal Your Gut,
and Have More Energy*

KUSHA KARVANDI, PES, CES, CSCS

Published by TCK Publishing

www.TCKPublishing.com

Get discounts and special deals on our best selling books at

www.tckpublishing.com/bookdeals

CONTENTS

About This Book

He who has health has hope. He who has hope has everything.

~ Arabic proverb

Most of my clients come to me with a goal to lose weight in specific areas. They want flat abs, tighter tummies, leaner legs, or less flabby arms. But they often don't think it's possible to quickly eliminate body fat in one particular area because that's what they've been told by previous coaches or what they've read in diet and exercise books.

I have seen my clients get the results they want faster than ever by using my individualized approach to help them become their own diet detectives and find which foods work best for their body. Now I want to share my individualized approach with you so you can have the body and confidence you desire.

What drives me crazy about the health and fitness industry is that it makes people think they are weak and that the best way to achieve the body they want is to suck it up and push harder.

Just look at popular TV shows like *The Biggest Loser* where trainers exhaust the participants with 8 hours of exercise per day and put them on extremely low calorie diets. But if more were better, why is it that the majority of these participants rebound and gain all their weight back – and then some?

The truth is, you're stronger than you think. It isn't that you somehow lack willpower or discipline, it's that you just don't yet have the right heuristic - which a mentor of mine once defined as:

the ability to make a decision based on limited information.

The beauty of a heuristic is that it doesn't drain your willpower the way calorie-counting or other fad diets can. In this book, I'll share with you how to craft your own diet heuristic so you can make good eating decisions no matter where you are or how much willpower you have.

The hardest part about getting in shape and losing weight is taking the first step. So don't worry if you've never been able to achieve your goal before. We tend to believe failure begets failure, but nearly all success stories begin with generous amounts of failure. If you've tried diets before that didn't work, don't worry because what I'm going to teach you isn't a diet – it's a way of thinking. With the right lens you'll be able to look at nutrition and fat loss differently, and make decisions that will get you results you can keep.

I know what you're thinking. This is just another quick fix gimmick. How could it be that one can eat flavorful, satiating foods and actually lose weight? Believe me, I thought the same thing when I began to study this concept. But what I found is that our bodies aren't programmed for obesity. Of course everyone has their own individual, natural set-point when it comes to weight. But when we began eating unnatural, processed foods, vegetables oils, and refined carbohydrates we shifted the nature of our body toward fat storage instead of fat burn.

In this book, I'm going to provide you with the tools to eat well while reaching your goals quickly. While your naysayers are counting calories, feeling deprived, and still struggling to lose weight, you'll be vibrant, full of energy, and supercharging your metabolism for sustained fat loss.

Eat Fat, Get Fit is for educational purposes only and is not intended to diagnose, treat, cure, or prevent any disease. Always consult with your healthcare professional before beginning a new diet or supplement regimen.

HOW THE BODY WORKS

ENERGY SYSTEMS

ATP – PC ENERGY PATHWAY

The ATP – PC energy pathway works to provide about ten seconds' worth of energy for activities such as sprints or heavy weight lifting. The benefit of this particular energy pathway or source is that it requires no oxygen and produces energy quickly.

How exactly does the pathway work?

As the name suggests, there are two components that play a role: ATP, known as Adenosine Triphosphate; and PC, known as Phosphocreatine.

ATP is the usable form of energy most commonly stored in muscle cells for muscular activities. Other forms of chemical energy – those absorbed from food – must be converted into ATP before the muscle cells can actually use them.

PC, at the same time, is stored in the muscle cells. When broken down, PC releases a significant amount of energy and part of that energy is used to resynthesize the ATP.

The storage of both ATP and PC is significantly small, however, which is why the ATP – PC energy pathway supplies only about 10 seconds' worth of energy.

As the body engages in physical activity and the energy capacity of the ATP and PC energy system is used up, the body will move on to either aerobic or anaerobic metabolism to continue with the creation of ATP (fuel).

Being aware of how your body uses the different types of energy found in a variety of foods will help you begin to make conscious decisions about the type of energy you consume at a given time of day. In this case, simple carbohydrates such as fruit would be ideal to consume 30 minutes before physical activity because of the body's ability to convert the fruit into usable energy quickly.

Coconut water is another excellent choice because it not only provides natural sugars but also blends the perfect balance of electrolytes.

THE ANAEROBIC METABOLIC PATHWAY

Better known as glycolysis (because it involves the breakdown of sugar), the anaerobic metabolic pathway leads to the breakdown of sugar to produce energy – the manufacturer of ATP from carbohydrates.

Glycolysis gives off energy through the partial breakdown of sugar without the need for oxygen. Similar to the ATP – PC energy pathway, it provides a quick supply of energy used in short and high-intensity bursts of activity. Each burst of energy lasts for only one to three minutes before the lactic acid accumulation reaches the lactate threshold.

When this threshold is reached, there is intense muscle pain, a burning sensation, and fatigue without the availability of another, alternate energy source.

Knowing that you are going to engage in short bursts of intense activity, such as weight training, you can plan ahead and select a snack or meal that will provide a good source of energy to support the anaerobic metabolic pathway – one that is relatively high in carbohydrates, such as brown rice or yams. Making a selection like this in anticipation of a certain type of activity will help your body be efficient about its energy usage.

AEROBIC METABOLISM

Aerobic metabolism provides most of the energy necessary for our daily activities, including physical activity that lasts more than one to three minutes. It is used primarily during less intense activities. It is also the fallback energy pathway for most endurance exercises.

A more complex system than the other two energy pathways, aerobic metabolism uses oxygen to convert protein, fats, and carbohydrates to ATP. The process for creating ATP via this method takes more time and relies on the body's circulatory system to transport oxygen to the working muscles.

A physically active person will generally move through these metabolic pathways as they exercise. When they begin their workout, anaerobic metabolism kicks in and produces ATP. As breathing becomes more rapid and the heart rate increases, more oxygen is available for aerobic metabolism.

Aerobic metabolism continues until the body reaches the lactate threshold. It is a cycle. When the body cannot take in oxygen fast enough, anaerobic metabolism will again take place to produce ATP.

Since the anaerobic system lasts only for a short time and lactic acid will likely build up over an extended period of anaerobic exercise, the intensity of such an activity cannot be maintained for long. Eventually you have to slow down and reduce the intensity of the activity, eliminating the buildup of lactic acid in the process.

Understanding this and knowing what is required for aerobic metabolism will help you better understand your body's needs during extended activity. Knowing that it is time to slow down, or even just knowing the importance of pacing the intensity of your activities to facilitate aerobic metabolism, will help you become more in tune with your body's functions and help you fuel your energy system more efficiently with healthier food choices.

Fats, specifically short- and medium-chain fatty acids such as milk fats and coconut oil, are best for this pathway. Short- and medium-chain fatty acids are absorbed much more efficiently than long-chain fatty acids such as olive oil and egg yolks. Short- and medium-chain fatty acids are transported directly to your liver, whereas long-chain fatty acids go through your lymphatic system.

In addition, short- and medium-chain fatty acids enjoy preferential oxidation. Optimizing fat oxidation is necessary to maintain a healthy weight and avoid ailments such as obesity and diabetes.

FUELING THE ENERGY SYSTEMS

ATP is developed based on a breakdown of nutrients contained in fuel. The key question, though, is what type of activity are you about to engage in and what fuel will best help your body generate energy efficiently?

Because it breaks down slowly, fat is the best fuel for endurance events. It is not, however, the best choice for high-intensity exercise. Anyone planning on sprinting, for example, or exercising at more than 50% of the maximum heart rate for their age, is better off with carbohydrates as their energy source. The body can break down carbohydrates faster than fats or proteins, making it ideal for high intensity, short duration activity.

Figure 1 on the next page summarizes the energy systems and the appropriate energy sources.

Figure 1

PRIMARY ENERGY SYSTEMS	DURATION OF ACTIVITY	BEST ENERGY SOURCE
ATP-PC	0-10 seconds	Carbohydrates
ATP-PC & Anaerobic Glycolysis	10-30 seconds	Carbohydrates
Anaerobic Glycolysis	30 sec-2 min	Carbohydrates
Anaerobic Glycolysis Aerobic Metabolism	2-3 min	Fats*
Aerobic Metabolism	3 minutes +	Fat

Depending on intensity

When you are exercising at a low intensity – below 50% of your maximum heart rate – you likely have enough stored fat to fuel your activity for hours, perhaps even days. The key to being able to function is oxygen. As long as you have sufficient oxygen to support fat metabolism, you can be active without needing to change your nutrient supply.

When comparing the appropriateness of fats and carbohydrates in energy production, remember that fats - especially saturated animal fats - are much more dense in fat-soluble vitamins and minerals than carbohydrates.

For athletes and those with labor-intensive jobs, a diet higher in carbohydrates is acceptable. But for most individuals whose lifestyles or professions are more sedentary, or who are just looking to lose body fat or gain muscle, they are better suited to a diet higher in fats with moderate carbohydrates and proteins.

With proper eating and appropriate physical training, these energy systems and pathways can become more efficient in providing energy to your body, allowing for extreme physical activities that last longer and have greater intensity.

FACTS ABOUT FAT

FACT #1: FAT WON'T MAKE YOU FAT

Many people still believe the fat you eat in food turns into fat on your body. Logical as it might sound, this notion is completely false. The fat in our food is fat we need to help our bodies function better. The fat we eat is not actually the same type of fat found in our bodies.

Keeping food diaries, journals, food logs, and counting calories are not long-term solutions to healthy eating or weight loss. These methods are, in fact, little more than a waste of paper and time. They can also seriously deprive you of the proper nutrition you need.

When you eat more fats, your body's ability to recognize satiety increases, and you learn to recognize when you are full. Many overweight and obese people do not eat enough of the right foods, which causes them to eat more of the wrong types of foods to satisfy their body's daily requirements.

FACT #2: MANY ESSENTIAL VITAMINS AND MINERALS COME FROM FATS

Most people don't know that fat has the highest density and best bioavailability of many essential minerals and vitamins. It affords the best absorption of key vitamins and minerals for most metabolic functions. It is no secret that a balanced diet should have the appropriate amounts of vitamins and minerals, both of which play major roles in the body's normal functions.

Deficiency of any of these vitamins and minerals can quickly lead to serious health problems.

FACT #3: FATS IMPROVE BLOOD SUGAR STABILITY

Unlike carbohydrates and proteins, fats will not cause your insulin to spike. This is crucial, especially when it comes to controlling moods and cravings.

A large release of insulin can cause weight gain and other diseases. An elevated level of insulin forbids your body to transform fat into energy.

FACT #4: FATS REDUCE CRAVINGS AND KEEP YOU FULL

Fat content in your diet can prevent you from eating too much. Fats release a hormone in the brain called cholecystokinin, or CCK. In addition to stimulating the digestion of fat and protein in the gastrointestinal system, CCK also acts as a hunger suppressant.

FACT #5: FATS OPTIMIZE HORMONE LEVELS

Fats help produce testosterone, cortisol, estrogen, and progesterone. These hormones are lipid soluble, meaning they are created from cholesterol and fat.

If your body fails to produce the proper amounts of these hormones, you may experience muscle atrophy, body fat storage, and diseases caused by hormonal imbalance. You can also experience a general lack of well-being, affecting your life and everyone around you.

THE REAL "BAD" FATS

Fat has been a controversial topic for decades and has generally earned a bad reputation. However, fats are as necessary to a healthy diet as other nutrients. Aside from being a great source of energy, fat helps the body absorb vitamins and is essential for blood clotting, muscle movement, and plays a vital role in our body's inflammatory response. The best fats are found in nuts, seeds, fish, and vegetables (monounsaturated and polyunsaturated fats). The worst kinds of fats, trans fats, have no known health benefits. Saturated fats, those found in animal fat and tropical oils, though bashed for years as "bad fat," are more beneficial to the body than previously believed. Each kind of fat serves a different purpose, and each should be moderated to meet an individual's needs.

Foods high in monounsaturated and polyunsaturated fats are better for the body, perhaps because they are more natural than trans fats. Monounsaturated fats are commonly found in olive oil, peanut oil, avocados, and most nuts. Polyunsaturated fats are commonly found in fatty fish, flaxseeds, and vegetable oils. Monounsaturated and polyunsaturated fats are more beneficial than trans fats, but polyunsaturated fats have less hydrogen atoms surrounding their carbon atoms (hence the term "unsaturated") which means they oxidize more easily in the body. Think of oxidation like rust in the body. Too much polyunsaturated fat can act like a firecracker for oxidation and inflammation in the tissues. Since the inception of refined, packaged foods, Americans have dramatically increased their consumption of polyunsaturated and trans fatty acids. These fats primarily come from unnatural vegetable oils (i.e. canola oil) and shortenings.

More saturated fats carry more fat-soluble vitamins. Thus, more good fats in the diet would (presumably) increase the absorption of fat-soluble nutrients. Saturated fats have been the most controversial type of fat. Since the 1950s, saturated fats have been characterized as "bad" because higher consumption of these fats is thought to be associated with a rise in blood cholesterol levels.

The issue has been researched for decades, but there is not enough evidence to confirm that saturated fats increase the risk of heart disease. In fact, clinical trials show that replacing animal fats with vegetable oils isn't as beneficial as people have been led to believe since the 1950s; it is likely that substituting saturated fats with polyunsaturated fats could promote cancer and maybe even heart disease. Current research also shows that saturated fats have been shown to actually protect against cancer.

Foods rich in trans fats are practically useless, and if not useless, are more harmful than beneficial. These fats have higher amounts of LDL cholesterol (bad cholesterol) and lower amounts of HDL cholesterol (good cholesterol). Higher consumption of trans fats can create inflammation which is connected to heart disease, stroke, diabetes, and other chronic conditions. It seems that trans fats deserve the blame that has been placed on saturated fats for the last half century.

Some of the best foods for the body are high in fats. Avocados are high in fat but are a great source of fiber and help to lower LDL cholesterol. Dark chocolate is high in fat, but studies show that those who eat it regularly are less likely to die from heart disease than those who do not. Eggs are high in fat but are also one of the most nutrient-dense foods; they are high in protein, loaded with vitamins, and great for losing weight. These foods, among many others, provide the perfect example for how generalizations about fat can affect healthy diet decisions in a bad way.

All in all, balance is the key to a complete diet. One person's nutritional needs can vary greatly from another's, and dietary needs change across your lifespan. Regardless of how good or bad certain fats are for the human body, no one element of a diet should outweigh the others. There is no exact formula to a balanced (and healthy) diet; everyone must listen to his or her own body.

FAT METABOLISM

THE FUNCTION OF THE LIVER

The liver is a vital organ with two very important functions. It filters toxins from the body and it helps metabolize fats.

The problem with this dual function, though, is that it isn't entirely practical. Like a person working two jobs, the liver cannot effectively focus on breaking down fats when it is busy and besieged with filtering toxins. In fact, when the liver is working overtime to remove toxins from the body, fat is being stored instead of metabolized.

To help your liver function properly, you need to choose the right foods, including foods that are toxin-free.

THE WORST IMPEDIMENTS TO FAT METABOLISM

To help our bodies metabolize fat properly, we need to make a list of the worst enemies of fat metabolism.

So, what are they?

- ARTIFICIAL SWEETENERS. To avoid overloading your body with toxins, you should avoid Splenda, sucralose, and aspartame. Stevia is okay.

- ALCOHOL. High levels of alcohol intake can cause serious liver problems and damage the organ that helps control fat metabolism. Minimal alcohol intake is recommended.

- PRESERVATIVES. These are unnatural and toxic to your body. Preservatives are found in almost all packaged goods.

- PESTICIDES. Be cautious about the types of fruits and vegetables you consume. Even organic fruits and vegetables can contain pesticides. Find a local CSA (Community Supported Agriculture) or farmer's market you trust. Use them as a source for your daily dose of pesticide-free fruits and vegetables.

- ARTIFICIAL ADDITIVES. Avoid MSG. Check the label and watch out for soy protein isolate and citric acid. Both of these additives produce MSG as a by-product. Many protein shakes and protein bars contain one or both of these additives and should therefore be avoided.

- TRANS FATS. Any products containing hydrogenated or even partially hydrogenated oils should be avoided.

- CORN SYRUP. Especially those with high fructose. They are often artificial and very high on the glycemic index, indicating that blood sugar levels can rise very quickly after ingesting.

- CAFFEINE. It is unnecessary to completely avoid caffeine, but you should limit your intake. Caffeine affects the body much the way carbohydrates do. Ingesting caffeine can cause blood sugar levels to rise and fall, resulting in the fat storage.

THE ROLE OF LEPTIN & GHRELIN

Leptin is a hormone that plays a major role in energy intake and expenditure, especially when it comes to appetite and fat metabolism. Leptin sends a signal to specific receptors of the hypothalamus, a part of the brain that regulates the body's hormones, to tell us if we are full or if we need to eat. When leptin is low, the brain senses famine and our appetite increases. When it is high, we feel full, satiated, and our metabolism kicks into high gear. Since leptin is produced by our adipose (fat) tissue, there is a directly proportional relationship between fat abundance and leptin abundance. So, you'd think that obese individuals would feel full all the time, right? Wrong.

The problem is that the receptors in the brain build up a tolerance and essentially become resistant to leptin when there is an overabundance. Conversely, when we crash diet or undergo liposuction or other extreme weight loss methods, our leptin levels plummet, leading to a spike in hunger and a corresponding drop in thyroid output and metabolic rate. Additionally, leptin levels are more sensitive to undereating than overeating. So, although you may feel a short-term boost in metabolism during a "diet," you inevitably crash by slowing down your metabolism.

Leptin levels are also tied to insulin levels, so they will normally increase right after you eat and when your body is storing energy (i.e., during sleep). This is why leptin dysfunction occurs with sleep deprivation as well as refined carbohydrate consumption. When you are sleeping, your body produces leptin so you rest instead of getting up to eat. When we disrupt our sleep cycle, it affects our leptin sensitivity and inevitably makes us leptin resistant. The same happens when we consume refined carbohydrates. Refined carbohydrates spike our insulin levels and lead to a corresponding surge in leptin levels. This overabundance of leptin will, again, lead to leptin resistance long term.

As our brains become more leptin resistant, they require more and more leptin for us to feel full. This is why we may sometimes feel like a bottomless pit or have uncontrollable cravings. When we begin to reduce our caloric intake, our bodies adjust by dropping leptin levels, spiking our appetite, and dropping energy levels and metabolic function. However, as we give our bodies time, they eventually adjust to the new lower levels of leptin and we reset our basal leptin levels. This is why gradually reducing consumption over time is far superior to crash dieting if you need to lose a significant amount of weight.

Besides excess weight, refined carbohydrates, and sleep deprivation, there are other culprits for leptin resistance. High stress levels, high toxicity of the body (including blood acidity), and even high-fructose diets can induce leptin resistance by impairing leptin's ability to cross the blood-brain barrier to reach the hypothalamus.

So what should you do? Don't crash diet. Instead, cut calories gradually and "cheat" once a week by having a calorie-heavy meal. This method of "cheating" helps reduce daily leptin levels without making your body feel starved or sense famine. Next, avoid high sugar and refined carbohydrate intake. Instead, eat more omega-3 fatty acids from sources such as fish, flaxseed, and walnuts.

Studies show that even when consumed at high caloric quantities, the body's leptin sensitivity increases when higher concentrations of omega-3 fatty acids are present. Also, avoid processed foods. Instead, increase your body's alkalinity by getting more fat-soluble vitamins and minerals (from high-quality animal fats), consuming vegetables (even if blended in a smoothie), and drinking lemon water and apple cider vinegar regularly.

Finally, make sure to sleep well and enough. Leptin levels naturally rise during our sleep cycles, so when we cut our sleep short, our body tries to correct this by decreasing leptin and increasing appetite. So sleeping for six hours or less on a regular basis will lead to lower daily levels of leptin and an obvious dysfunction with normal hormonal balance and cravings.

Another hormone, **ghrelin**, plays a similar role. Ghrelin is secreted by the stomach lining when our stomachs are empty. It then sends a signal to the brain and crosses the same blood-brain barrier as leptin to reach the hypothalamus which triggers our hunger mechanism. When we eat, ghrelin levels drop to lower hunger. So when we overeat or crash diet, we create dysfunction which, again, disrupts our metabolism and hunger control systems. Just one more unequivocal reason to avoid the extreme ends of the consumption spectrum and the mythical "silver bullet" to weight management.

WHY WE CRAVE

RECOGNIZING AND OVERCOMING FOOD ADDICTIONS

The following scenario is common to many people. You are in a grocery store and you see a chocolate bar. You want to get one, but you are fighting the urge to buy it. Or, it is after dinner, you have just eaten, and you are already full. The problem, of course, is that you crave something sweet.

We all have these cravings and we try very hard to fight them, but they often feel impossible to resist. Most people crave the refined carbohydrates (sugar and wheat) found in cookies, bread, cakes, brownies, candies, donuts, bagels, and ice cream. Many people who want to lose weight are caught up in this fundamental battle to conquer their cravings.

In his book *How We Get Fat*[1], author Gary Taubes explains how we can control cravings by cutting foods from our diet that elevate our insulin levels, such as sweets and starches. When we ingest sweets and starches that are high on the glycemic index, meaning they cause a rapid rise in blood sugar, our body compensates by producing large amounts of insulin and stress hormones. Not only does this lead to fat storage, but as our blood sugar level begins to rapidly decline, we crave the same substances to spike them again.

THE BRAIN AND CRAVINGS

According to Julia Ross, author of *The Mood Cure,*[2] food cravings originate in the brain. Chemicals in our brain regulate thoughts and obsessions about food. False signals to the brain, created by eating processed foods, can initiate cravings for certain foods even when a person is not actually hungry.[3]

Your brain creates an impulse that is extremely difficult to ignore and essentially takes control of your body. Hungry or not, you eat foods to satisfy the craving.

As explained by Ross, cravings often occur because processed foods are deficient in specific amino acids necessary to regulate the functions that can affect both mood and cravings. There is an amino acid called DL-Phenylalanine (DLPA), which is a form of phenylalanine. If you are particularly affected by cravings, one of the suggested solutions is to take a supplement with amino acids like DLPA, which works as an appetite suppressant and can thus eliminate the need to act on cravings.[4]

MOOD AND AMINO ACIDS

Amino acids are the building blocks of protein in our bodies. They are also essential for the central nervous system to function properly. They act as neurotransmitters or as precursors to these neurotransmitters, helping to receive and send messages through the brain. In fact, the transmission of messages may go wrong if amino acids including protein and L-tryptophan are not present together.

Several diseases and other disorders can occur if amino acid intake is inadequate or if there is an inability to digest proteins. Severe symptoms of this deficiency include ADD, depression, anxiety, and several other mental disorders; a more common symptom is severe cravings.

If a person is low in the amino acid L-tryptophan, they may have cravings for carbohydrates, alcohol, or drugs. L-tryptophan is necessary for producing serotonin, a natural anti-depressant. If you are low in endorphins, your brain may induce cravings for sweets and other simple carbohydrates. The amino acid DLPA will also help reduce these comfort-food cravings, but only temporarily.

Ross advocates the use of L-tryptophan and other amino acids as behavioral-change catalysts and not long-term solutions, although most are safe to be taken long-term. Instead, she advises a change in diet, one rich in amino acids commonly found in high-quality animal products.[5]

THE EFFECTS OF GLUTEN

A protein called gluten can be found in several grains including wheat, rye, spelt, and barley, which for some people can be very hard to digest. Unfortunately, most treats people crave are made from gluten grains and can become quite addictive.

In his book *Dangerous Grains*,[6] Dr. James Braly explains why some cravings come from the body's inability to digest gluten properly. According to the research he cites, undigested partial proteins, or peptides, have morphine-like substances that become similar to addictive drugs once inside the bloodstream.

Due to the pleasant and relaxing feeling these potent foods cause, many people unconsciously develop cravings for these types of foods and become addicted to them as they give in to the cravings.[7]

DIS-EASE IN THE GUT

"Disease begins in the colon."

This aphorism has become a stable conclusion for many healthcare professionals because of the overwhelming evidence showing that imbalance in the growth of bacteria, parasites, and candida in the colon can cause nutritional- or dietary-based issues.

The cause of most colon-based diseases, however, is what we consume. For example, certain products, when introduced in the body, produce an overgrowth of fungi, bad bacteria, and yeast inside the body. The causes of this buildup can include antibiotics and processed foods, both of which destroy the good bacteria necessary to maintain a balance of bacteria in the body.

This imbalance can often cause disease because it compromises the digestive system. Good bacteria, which aid in the digestion and absorption of nutrients, can be destroyed by the overgrowth of bad bacteria, which thrive off processed sugar and carbohydrates, leading to continued cravings. Parasites may also exist in the body, attacking good bacteria and consuming sugar.

Dr. Natasha Campbell-McBride explains how "a craving for sweet and starchy food is typical for all people with abnormal bodily flora, particularly [those] with candida overgrowth." Studies show that things such as birth control pills and excessive sugar can encourage the growth of bad bacteria. Other common causes of cravings include the following:

DIET LOW IN SATURATED FAT

A diet low in fat cannot satisfy hunger. Many people report feelings of continued hunger after eating a low-fat meal. In *Eat Fat Lose Fat*[8] by Sally Fallon and Mary Enig, PhD, the authors state that saturated fats are necessary for the nerves, brain, hormones, immune system, and metabolism to function at a high level of efficiency.

Fallon and Enig also explain that saturated fats, at appropriate levels, can help give the body a feeling of satiety, making us feel content and full.

When we consume healthy fats, such as those found in raw cream, raw butter, raw nuts, organic eggs, and the meat from grass-fed animals, our body releases a hormone that tells us we are full and have eaten enough.

In his book *The Fourfold Path to Healing*,[9] Dr. Tom Cowan explains how "our brain is specifically designed to sense the fat content of our food and to tell us to stop eating when the proper amount of fat has been ingested. When the need for fats and the nutrients they contain is satisfied, we stop eating. The body's requirement for fats is so great, and the appetite that spurs the body to obtain those fats is so strong, that binge eating is likely to occur if fats are omitted from regular meals."[10]

LOW VITAMIN B LEVELS

Undigested waste may be in your intestinal tract if you have been consuming refined and processed foods. More specifically, grains that did not undergo the traditional processes of soaking and fermenting may become blocked in your body, and your body may start to breed too much bad bacteria and not enough good bacteria to maintain the right balance.

Of course, it would be hard for your intestines to absorb the essential B vitamins under these conditions. The brain needs B6 to make serotonin, a neurotransmitter important in the promotion of a general state of well-being, happiness, and satisfaction.

LOW-CALORIE DIETING

Low-calorie dieting can cause brain nutrition deficiency or the "dieter's malnutrition." Julia Ross determines this to be a primary cause of food cravings.[11]

Less food is needed to satisfy the basic nutrient needs if, and only if, the body digests vital nutrients efficiently. With this proper assimilation, there is also a lasting feeling of satiety. On the other hand, if a person does not digest and absorb nutrients properly, or if they do not consume sufficient nutrient-dense foods, the body's natural reaction is to ask for more food because it needs more nutrients to live.

Although modern processed foods are high in calories, Dr. Cowan explains, they have very low levels of nutrients. While it may satisfy the appetite, the satisfaction only lasts for a short time. The body continuously sends signals to the brain that it needs to eat more to absorb the nutrients the body requires.[12]

SUGAR, SUGAR, SUGAR

Research shows that consuming large amounts of sugar can make a person crave more of it.

Nora Gedgaudas, CNS, CNT, explains that if a person consumes high quantities of starch and sugar, their brain and body can become accustomed to, or metabolically adapted to, burning glucose instead of fat for fuel.

Many people who consume sugary breakfasts, such as cereals and breakfast bars, often feel hungry in as little as an hour. This results in continued sweet cravings. People may even feel ill if they are not consuming a constant stream of sugar-based foods. The science behind this sugary habit is that processed carbohydrates are absorbed by our body faster. They produce an unnaturally rapid rise in blood glucose, putting the body in a state of shock.

This results in the body quickly producing large quantities of insulin. An overproduction of insulin can eventually lead to a sudden decline of blood glucose.

Once the blood sugar level fluctuates, it can trigger cravings, mood swings, migraines, drowsiness, weak spells, and other serious health conditions. In the long term, this can even lead to Type 2 Diabetes.

FOOD ADDITIVES

Manufacturers sometimes mix chemicals into their processed food products for a variety of reasons. Some foods, like cookies and cereals, actually contain addictive ingredients that will cause you to eat and crave more.

Processed foods are considered junk foods that often contain chemicals and preservatives that negatively affect the formation of neurotransmitters. Experts agree that these food additives can have a direct effect on the human brain. A change in diet can actually solve this problem of addiction.

But more than just cravings, these toxins and chemicals found in processed foods can cause alterations in our hormones and our inherent slimming abilities. Studies expose that the higher the levels of these chemicals and toxins in the body, the higher the occurrence of body fat storage and even obesity.

ALLERGIES

It is not uncommon that the foods people are unknowingly allergic to are also the same foods they crave. When someone craves a particular food such as wheat, which is a common food allergen, more often than not they may have a mild allergy to wheat.

Unfortunately, it is easy for people to yearn for that compensatory feeling of comfort and happiness and overlook a potential allergy that may be causing symptoms such as fatigue, mood fluctuation, inflammation, and fat storage.

If you are experiencing abnormal and intense cravings for a specific unhealthy food type, it may be a good idea to have your doctor run an allergy test.

STRESSED ENDOCRINE SYSTEMS AND HORMONES

Bruce Rind, MD, an expert in adrenal and thyroid health, avers that sick and weakened adrenals can also be a cause for cravings.

With an unhealthy thyroid and adrenals, a person may crave grains, sweets, salt, or even combinations of these. Eating a low-fat diet, having weak fat metabolism, and not getting enough cholesterol and fat-soluble vitamins like vitamin A can contribute to weak adrenals. Mercury and other toxins can also be causes of unhealthy and damaged adrenal functions. These toxins, as mentioned earlier, can severely damage the human body by disrupting the hormones.

Together with a poor diet, imbalanced hormones can increase cravings and lead to other health problems.

NUTRITIONAL DEFICIENCIES

The Story of Dr. Weston Andrew Price

During the 1930s, Dr. Weston Price was practicing dentistry in Cleveland, Ohio. One day he noticed that healthy people had better teeth, gums, and jaws than those who were not healthy. Based on his findings, Weston concluded that the foundation of true health is based on what we eat.[13]

Dr. Price became well known for his theories and for essentially establishing the relationship between nutrition, physical health, and dental health. He studied what people were eating and identified the underlying dietary and lifestyle causes of decay and damage to the teeth, jaw, and gums. He also theorized that the general decline in dental health could well be the result of the growing number of processed foods in the average person's diet.

In search of answers, Dr. Price retired from dentistry to travel the world. He met with several indigenous people who did not have access to processed food and examined their teeth. As a result of his work, which took him from Africa to Alaska and from the Swiss Alps to the Polynesian islands, he became known as the "Charles Darwin of Nutrition" and the "Father of Preventive Dentistry."

In total, he studied 14 different tribes, looking to determine factors that contributed to oral health.

His research showed that people tended to have fewer cavities the farther away they lived from "civilization." In other words, the more primitive the people's mode of living was, the healthier their teeth. The farther away he got from the civilized world, the less decay he found, and the healthier people were. The people were so healthy that in some cultures, they were even unfamiliar with cancer and heart disease.

He uncovered a wide variety of diets as he considered evidence of dental health and the factors that appeared to promote it. Compared with the diets of a civilized population, all the diets he discovered supplied at least four times the amount of water-soluble vitamins and minerals, and at least ten times the amount of fat-soluble vitamins.

Another discovery Dr. Price made was that the parents in these indigenous tribes, both father and mother, held to strict premarital and preconception nutritional regimens. The mothers' and fathers' good health helped to produce healthy babies. Children were also born several years apart, giving the mother time to recuperate and recover after each pregnancy.

Dr. Price's study also found that pregnant or lactating women were kept as healthy as possible with special diets created to keep them at the top of their health.

Unfortunately, though, Dr. Price's study showed that just a generation of separation from these indigenous diets was enough to cause a sharp rise in health problems. There were crowded teeth requiring wisdom teeth extraction, issues with reduced immunity, and a variety of degenerative diseases.

Notice how record numbers of Americans today are suffering from heart disease, obesity, diabetes, food allergies, and cancer. Native Americans, on the other hand, were once strong and healthy simply from living off the resources of the land.

In his book, *Nutrition and Physical Degeneration*,[14] Dr. Price presents his findings along with some photographs that show the striking differences between healthy individuals and those just a generation behind them.

The invention of "innovations" known as processed foods may actually not be the greatest discovery for humans. Instead of making lives easier, processed food has destroyed the health of many.

Five decades after his death, many have yet to take notice of Dr. Price's work in which he suggested a nutrient-dense, whole, organic diet for healthier teeth and a healthier body.

Many experts, however, are now looking into dental amalgams and root canals as a cause of poor health and trigger for disease. Holistic dentistry has become more popular as more people have started to see the connection between diet, dental health, and general health.

ANIMAL FOOD ESSENTIALS

Dr. Price assessed the importance of eating animal-based food when he traveled to the South Sea Islands of the Pacific. He initially hoped to discover plants, fruits, and vegetables that might be able to supply the body with all the vitamins and nutrients needed for health and growth, even without animal products.

Ultimately, however, he failed. He found that no such plant existed.

Vegetarians are susceptible to several vitamin deficiencies, including deficiencies in vitamin D, A, K2, B6, B12, as well as deficiencies in cholesterol, zinc, essential fatty acids, and, conditionally, essential amino acids.

Most of these vitamins and minerals are found naturally in meat or animal products. Deficiencies of these nutrients can result in several problems including anemia, rickets, poor growth, neuromuscular deficits, and even blindness.

Dr. Price found a group of people on the island of Viti Levu who were relying largely on plant products yet ate shellfish at least once every few months. They traded the plants and fruits they harvested from the mountains for shellfish caught by coast-dwelling groups.

Incredibly dense in animal-based nutrients, one serving of shellfish per month can give you the same amount of vitamin B12 as two servings of salmon a week. Likewise, a single serving of oysters or clams per week can provide an equal amount of zinc as can a quarter pound of beef eaten per day.

People who plan to eat fewer animal products will benefit greatly by adding a small amount of shellfish to their diet for proper nutrition. For those allergic to or who don't care for shellfish, the amount of animal products needed to be consumed might be higher than suggested.

Dr. Price's research led him to the following conclusions about vegetarianism. First, he failed to find even one group of primitive racial stock that had formed and grown excellent healthy bodies by eating only vegetables, fruits, and other plant foods. Second, he found traces of degeneration in the form of atypical dental arches on those people who were long under this system. This degeneration was much more pronounced than those primitive groups that were not following the same plant-based diet.

Dr. Price's study came with the definitive conclusion that, for a healthier and stronger body, animal products should be eaten throughout childhood and into adulthood. Animal products such as liver, egg yolks, shellfish, bone broth, and dairy products are the richest in vitamins and minerals.[15]

Every person needs to learn and understand their own body and how to take care of it. They must understand how to properly nourish their bodies by supplying them with all the vitamins and minerals needed, even if this means abandoning a particular lifestyle or set of beliefs. It is only natural that we consume animal products to get essential nutrients in adequate quantities.

CORRUPTION IN THE FOOD PROCESSING INDUSTRY

Vital nutrients and enzymes, in particular those needed to break down fats in the body, are not present in non-organic animal fats such as chicken, pork, and eggs. This is most likely because they are inadequately fed and poorly raised.

For convenience and affordability, the modern food industry has implemented poor production practices to mass-produce dairy products. These include the following:

Feeding grains to cows. Cows should eat grass to ingest the proper vitamins and minerals they need. Forcing cows to eat grains that are not found in their natural habitat can cause them to become sick and unhealthy and produce unhealthy by-products in their milk and meat.

Giving antibiotics to cows. It is uncommon for a free-range, grass-fed cow to become sick and require antibiotics. However, modern farming practices keep cows confined to tighter spaces and they are fed grain instead of grass. These two conditions commonly cause the cows to get sick, potentially leading to a prescription for antibiotics. In addition, many farms will commonly give antibiotics to their entire cow stock as a cost effective preventative measure. These antibiotics can end up in the products we consume.

Injecting hormones into the cows to increase their ability to produce milk and offspring. These hormones are unnatural. Similar to antibiotics, these too can be passed on to the consumer.

Meat and dairy products from grain-fed cows lack some of the most essential vitamins, minerals, and enzymes necessary for our body's health. The products from grain-fed cows are missing two particularly important enzymes: the lactase enzyme and the lipase enzyme. The lactase enzyme is necessary to properly digest milk, while the lipase enzyme is needed to break down fats so they are not stored as body fat.

Conversely, meat from grass-fed cows has vital vitamins, minerals, omega-6 fats, omega-3 fats, and CLA (conjugated linoleic acid). Grass-fed cows naturally produce organic, unpasteurized, and unhomogenized dairy products that have several benefits.

These products have a perfect balance of omega-3 and omega-6 fats for a healthy body. Only a few types of food have this perfect balance.

Milk products from grass-fed cows have five times more CLA than those from grain-fed cows. CLA is one of the most potent cancer-fighting foods. CLA can also aid in fat metabolism. This is abundant in grass-fed products.

Compared to grain-fed products, meat and dairy from grass-fed cows have a significantly higher amount of beta-carotene, vitamin A, vitamin D, and vitamin E.

Dairy from grass-fed animals is significantly higher in calcium and protein.

These products are free from antibiotics and hormones that can be unknowingly ingested by the consumer.

They are a natural, great food option to burn fat and build muscle.

Raw organic dairy takes longer to spoil.

For those with cow's milk allergies, goat products can be an excellent alternative. Goat products typically come from grass-fed goats and provide the same essential fat-soluble vitamins and minerals.

When purchasing lamb, look for the New Zealand sources, as they are more likely to have come from an ethical, high-quality producer.

INTERPRETING THE FOOD LABEL

It is always best to check the nutrition label of the products you purchase. Understanding what is written on the label can help you tremendously, but it takes some effort. Here are a few tips to summarize the above information:

If you see soy protein isolate and citric acid on the label, don't buy it. These two create MSG as a by-product in their manufacturing process. The truth is, most companies don't include MSG in their labels, knowing this is something people try to avoid; instead, they list these two names that seem harmless to the average person.

Don't be mistaken. Ascorbic acid is not the same as vitamin C, although it is a component of vitamin C. Consider instead products with acerola, which is a natural source of complete vitamin C.

Search for sucralose in the label even if the label says sugar-free or aspartame-free. Sucralose is barely better than aspartame. Go natural and choose products with stevia. Stevia has zero effect on blood sugar and contains no calories. Moreover, it does not negatively affect fat metabolism.

Avoid hydrogenated and even partially hydrogenated oils. After World War II, producing highly unsaturated oils from soybeans and corn became possible. Processors were allowed to selectively hydrogenate the types of fatty acids that have three double bonds found in soy and canola oil. The new method was dubbed partial hydrogenation.

Partial hydrogenation allowed processors to replace cottonseed oil with more unsaturated soybean and corn oils in shortenings and margarines. Contrary to popular belief, because of this process and the high quantity of trans fats, margarine is very unhealthy and should be avoided. Currently, soybean oil dominates the market and is used in approximately 80% of all hydrogenated oils.

The specific combination of fatty acids found in soybean oil results in shortenings that hold almost 40% trans fat, an increase of around 5% over cottonseed oil and roughly 15% over corn oil. Processed and produced from a hybrid form of rapeseed, canola oil is predominantly rich in fatty acids that contain the three double bonds and the shortening can contain as much as 50% trans fats. Although not indicated on labels for the liquid oil, trans fats can be also formed during the deodorization of canola oil.

Only consume traditional and natural fats. Foods made from vegetable oil should be avoided (with the exception of olive oil), especially when they are produced from vegetables that are not naturally oily. Instead of margarine, it is recommended that you use organic butter from grass-fed cows when cooking or preparing meals.

Avoid high-fructose corn syrup. High-fructose corn syrup and corn syrup are immensely artificial and high glycemic, meaning they cause a rapid spike in blood sugar. These can eventually lead to fat storage as well.

Agave is also highly processed. It can be similar to high-fructose corn syrup in how the body metabolizes it. Do not be fooled by the claims of natural variance between light and dark agave. The dark agave is actually just an erroneously burned or overly cooked light agave.

AVOID AGAVE

Food sweeteners are a much debated topic in the world of diet and nutrition. Whether you eat all natural and organic foods or live mainly on quick-fix meals, you may have heard the controversy about added sweeteners. Many people are on the lookout for a sweetener that is low-calorie or low on the glycemic index, without sacrificing taste. Recent years have brought about a focus on natural sweeteners that are less processed than the widely used high fructose corn syrup. Agave nectar was created in the 1990s and has since become one of the more controversial sweeteners available due to the long running debate about whether it's good or bad for your health.

Agave nectar, which comes from the native Mexican agave plant, is often labeled as all-natural, raw, and organic, but is it healthier for the body than cane sugar? The sweetener debate will likely go on for many years as new "natural" sweeteners are found, but the truth about agave syrup is out. This truth will disturb many who thought they had found a natural alternative to cane sugar. One of the most disturbing facts about agave nectar is that many of the common products on grocery store shelves are very similar to the high fructose corn syrup they're trying to avoid.

Another concern about this sweetener is the way it is made. Agave nectar most commonly found in grocery stores is highly processed in much the same way as high fructose corn syrup. While some people do make a sweetener from agave that is minimally processed by simply boiling agave sap, this is not what is found in the grocery aisle. Commercially available agave nectar is made from the root of the plant, which is very starchy. This process makes for a sweetener that is very high in fructose, giving it a similar makeup to high fructose corn syrup. This concentrated fructose product, in both agave nectar and HFCS, doesn't occur anywhere in nature and can only be made by man.

Agave nectar does have a low glycemic index which is one of the main reasons it has become so popular. Some people with diabetes think they can use this sweetener when they can't use others. The reason for this idea is that fructose is processed by the liver, rather than the intestine, leading to the claim that diabetics can use agave nectar. But once processed, fructose inhibits the hormones in the body that tell you you're full. This often leads to weight gain and makes the body hold onto excess fat.

Due to the outstanding evidence against agave nectar, and the complicated way in which it is made, it is best for everyone to limit their use of this product. Agave syrup is no more of a natural product than HFCS and can even lead to overeating and weight gain. Those who are looking for a sweetener can seek other, less processed, alternatives like honey or maple syrup. These options are as close to nature as you can get and they offer a satisfactory level of sweetness to most foods.

AVOID CARRAGEENAN

Carrageenan is primarily seen in processed foods and drinks, including almond, coconut, and soy milk. It is used for retaining moisture, binding, and contributing to the thickness of the mixture. Some studies show that degraded carrageenan can cause severe ulcerations in the gastrointestinal tract and in some cases, gastrointestinal cancer.

BE WARY OF GOITROGENIC FOODS

Many milk alternatives such as almond milk may seem harmless, but almond milk not only contains large amounts of sugar it is also a goitrogenic food that contains chemicals harmful to the thyroid.

Goitrogenic toxins are typically produced from almonds when soaked in water. This water is commonly used to produce almond milk. Goitrogenic toxins should be avoided as these can cause low thyroid function and contribute to the development of a goiter, or swelling of the thyroid gland.

Consuming a moderate amount of almond milk daily has not proven to be an imminent danger to people with healthy thyroids. However, for those with an already unhealthy thyroid, the risk can be significant.

GLUTEN-FREE

If produced properly, ordinary breads made with wheat are highly valuable for our health. With today's mass production, however, and manufacturing malpractices, the quality of bread has seriously declined.

Gluten is used to hold moisture and bind food. It can damage the lining of the small intestine, negatively affecting the absorption of nutrients, leading to serious malnutrition and associated diseases.

Although it also contains gluten, sourdough bread is a better alternative as it can easily be broken down. It is actually lower on the glycemic index than wheat bread, meaning it raises blood sugar more slowly and is less likely to induce the stress responses associated with fat storage.

If you are interested in making your own bread, below is a list of great gluten-free ingredients to try:

First, you must choose two of these **grainy** or **crumbly** flours:

- Coconut
- Rice
- Corn
- Amaranth
- Millet

Add **binding flour**. You can choose one of these:

- Arrowroot
- Pea or Pulse Flour
- Tapioca Flour
- Buckwheat
- Potato Starch

Mix in one to two of these **binders** as well:

- Guar Gum
- Egg
- Sago
- Flaxseed gel

For flavor, texture, and lower carbohydrates, include one to two of these ingredients

- Ground Flaxseed
- Ground Sesame Seeds
- Ground Almonds
- Ground Crispy Nuts

THE ROLE OF OSTEOCALCIN IN FAT LOSS

Osteocalcin is an important bone-building protein found in bone and dentin. It is also thought to participate in regulating the body's metabolic process. Osteocalcin depends on vitamin K2 (which is synergistic with vitamin D) to add carbon dioxide in a process called carboxylation. Studies found that undercarboxylated osteocalcin promotes a leaner body by stimulating the production of testosterone and insulin.

Recent literature suggests that osteocalcin deficient mice used in a study were fatter and had higher blood glucose. They simply did not burn energy at a high enough rate. Giving these mice uncarboxylated osteocalcin led to an improved insulin secretion and glucose tolerance. An improvement in insulin secretion tends to correlate with weight loss because the body is better able to regulate hormones and the metabolic process.

Evidence at this point is inconclusive as to whether undercarboxylated osteocalcin is responsible for producing a testosterone-boosting and fat-burning effect on the human body, although based on clinical studies, there seems to be a general concurrence that it might play a role.

It has been shown that those with vitamin K deficiency – and, therefore, low blood glucose tolerance – can take vitamin K2 supplements in order to improve their insulin and glucose metabolism. This could potentially help with weight loss in humans.

Vitamins A and D also play a role. Healthy levels of vitamins A and D are also necessary for bone health. Vitamin K works to regulate carboxylation and vitamin D stimulates transcription of osteocalcin. The degree to which carboxylation is experienced in humans is based on how much vitamin K (as well as vitamins A and D) are present in the daily diet. Human beings can be deficient in vitamins K, A, and D due to dietary choices and/or various physical disorders or diseases, such as autoimmune disorders.

Increased undercarboxylated osteocalcin levels seem to correlate with a reduction in serum glucose, which is something that can result after physical exercise. Therefore, it can be assumed that a combination of physical exercise and an appropriate amount of vitamins A, D, and K in the diet can work together to stimulate insulin production and promote fat loss through the metabolic process.

Genetic evidence reveals that a genetic defect in men with testicular dysfunction could be responsible for glucose intolerance and excessive weight. This could mean that undercarboxylated osteocalcin actually acts as a hormone in human beings. Although evidence is currently inconclusive on this subject, there is reason to believe that, like mice used in studies of undercarboxylated osteocalcin, this protein is hormonally active.

This leads to the question of whether we should have a vitamin K deficiency, since vitamin K limits the circulation of undercarboxylated osteocalcin throughout the body. Answers here are also rather inconclusive. The body needs vitamin K for certain metabolic processes, and vitamin K supplements enhance poor performance of insulin and glucose performance in human test subjects. Having a sufficient amount of vitamin K (as well as vitamins D and A) in the body is ideal for regulating metabolic processes.

THE GENETICS OF GLUTEN SENSITIVITY

One of two genes, HLA-DQ2 or HLA-DQ8, is commonly present in people with celiac disease. These and several other HLA-DQ genes heighten the risk for non-celiac gluten sensitivity. The HLA-DQ genes are what determine if our body can or cannot detect gluten, including whether the type of gluten is harmless or harmful to our body.

To recognize gluten as a harmful invader, the immune system must be triggered to see patterns that are quite similar to an infection. There are different answers for different people, for example:

Some people may have unidentified genes that can cause the immune system to consider an undigested fragment of the gluten protein as a foreign invader.

Some may have dysbiosis or damaged gut flora, which they may have developed from using antibiotics or eating food that is not easily digested. With this, the immune system may recognize the undigested gluten fragment as a microbial invader from the dysbiosis.

A nutrient-deficient diet can also interfere with the body's capacity to block immune cells from attacking harmless proteins. TGF-beta is a chemical the body uses to block immune cells. TGF- beta is stronger with vitamin A. If your diet is vitamin-A deficient, your body's ability to keep its immune system from attacking harmless proteins like gluten is compromised.

The following is a list of typical consumer items that may unexpectedly contain gluten so it is important to check the ingredients:

- Tomato and spaghetti sauces
- Prepackaged rice or pasta
- Vegetable cooking sprays
- Veined cheeses like Roquefort and blue
- Condensed canned soups
- Instant coffees and teas (flavored)
- Chow mein noodles
- Bouillon cubes or powdered gravy and other sauce mixes
- Artificial coffee creamer
- Ground spices
- Seafood product imitations
- Communion wafers
- Chewing gum

The list below points to label ingredients that can indicate the presence of gluten:

- Hydrolyzed plant protein (HPP)
- Hydrolyzed vegetable protein (HVP)
- Modified food starch (source is either corn or wheat)

- Mustard powder (some contain gluten)
- Monosodium glutamate (MSG)
- Gelatinized starch
- Natural flavoring, fillers
- Whey protein concentrate
- Whey sodium caseinate
- White vinegar or white grain vinegar
- Rice malt (contains barley or koji)
- Rice syrup (contains barley enzymes)
- Dextrin, malt, maltodextrin

THE ILLUSION OF ORGANIC

Pesticides are toxins that can often contaminate organic soil via local runoff from non-organic farms. Large corporations are constantly looking to use the term "organic" more freely. One of the major culprits is big box stores. Many products may say "organic" on the label but may not technically be organic because of the above-mentioned run off from non-organic farms.

If you want to find uncontaminated organic food such as fresh fruits and vegetables, go to your local Community Supported Agriculture (CSA) or other farmer's market. The products here are organically farmed and carefully checked. To find a local CSA check out: www.localharvest.org/csa [16]

CORNUCOPIA.ORG

Founded by Mark Kastel and Will Fantle, the Cornucopia Institute engages in several activities that support the ecological ideologies underlying sustainable and organic farming. The Cornucopia Institute conducts comprehensive studies and thorough investigations on issues regarding agriculture. It provides useful information to agriculturists, farmers, and, most important, to consumers.

The website **www.cornucopia.org** offers scorecards that help consumers make better buying decisions. On the site, you can view a complete list of brands for some of the most common food products, including cereal, eggs, and dairy, to name a few. The lists include the brand information, organic status, and a rating that will identify the product's quality.[17]

WHY PALEO DIETS ARE FLAWED

Among the popular diet fads is the Paleo Diet. Although there are key lessons we can learn from our Paleolithic ancestors, the current diet fad purports a few myths you must understand:

MYTH 1: *Our Paleolithic ancestors ate large quantities of meat, which they evolved to consume.*

TRUTH: We have no known genetic, physiological, or anatomical adaptations to meat consumption. In fact, we actually have many adaptations to plant consumption. Unlike carnivores that can naturally manufacture their own vitamin C from eating meat, our ancestors had to get vitamin C through plant consumption. We also have a longer digestive tract than carnivores because the food we eat needs to stay in our bodies longer to give the plant matter more time to digest. In terms of teeth, as omnivores we have large molars, which were designed to break down fibrous plant tissue. We do not have carnassials, which are the teeth that carnivores have to shred meat. We did have adaptations to animal consumption, but that was specifically to milk, not meat. This does not mean humans should avoid meat, it just means that we did not "evolve" as a species to predominantly consume meat.

MYTH 2: *Paleolithic people did not eat whole grains or legumes.*

TRUTH: Our ancestors developed stone tools 30,000 years ago (before the invention of agriculture) for grinding up seeds and grain. There is also evidence in the fossils of Paleolithic people's teeth to prove this myth is inaccurate.

MYTH 3: *Paleo foods are the only foods Paleolithic people ate.*

TRUTH: Almost all the foods recommended by Paleo Diet books are domesticated products. They did not have access to foods like olive oil because machinery is required to extract the oil. Other examples include apricots, almonds, carrots, and bananas, all of which modern civilization altered to make their consumption possible through advanced agricultural hybridization.

The reality of this diet fad is that there is no one paleo diet. There are numerous Paleolithic diets based on the local available resources.

The main things to take away here are:

- There was regional and seasonal variability in true Paleolithic diets.
- Our Paleolithic ancestors ate meat, but they also ate the organs and bone marrow.
- Lessons we can learn from our Paleolithic ancestors:
- No one diet is correct; diversity is key in order to get all the essential vitamins, minerals, and enzymes we need.
- We need to eat fresh food over packaged foods. Foods full of preservatives have a negative effect on our natural gut flora and good gastrointestinal bacteria. Consuming whole, unprocessed foods provides our bodies with the necessary fiber for proper digestion and blood sugar production.[18]

NUTRITIONAL PRODUCTS

DIETARY SUPPLEMENTS FOR ALL GOALS

WATER

Water may not be your typical supplement but water is, in fact, the most important nutrient of the body. It helps in digestion and is heavily involved in several bodily functions, significant for all metabolic functions.

Ideally, you should drink half your body weight in fluid ounces per day. On days you workout and exercise, you should add 20 ounces for every pound of body weight lost during your workout through perspiration (e.g., a 180 lb man who loses 1 lb of water through perspiration during a workout should drink 110 ounces of water that day).

PROBIOTICS AND PRO-GUT FLORA

Probiotics are needed for a clean intestinal tract and optimal nutrient absorption. The refrigerated brands are strongly recommended.

Start with a minimum of 1 to 3 billion parts per capsule, and based on how you feel, gradually make your way to consuming 40 billion parts per capsule.

Probiotics can also be found in many naturally fermented foods and many organic foods, including Kombucha tea, sourdough, natural sauerkraut, kefir, yogurt, microalgae, miso soup, tempeh, pickles, and kimchi.

CLA

CLA, or conjugated linoleic acid, is a fatty acid primarily found in meats and dairy. CLA can improve body composition by reducing body fat and increasing lean body mass. The best sources of CLA are raw organic dairy products, grass-fed beef, lamb, and flax seed. It is best to use three to four grams per day.

OMEGA-3 FATTY ACIDS

Omega-3 fatty acids are commonly found in marine and plant oils. Considered vital fatty acids, omega-3 fatty acids are important for normal metabolism. The best sources are cod liver oil or fish oil capsules from Atlantic salmon. It is recommended that you use 1000 mg per day, which is 500 mg of EPA and 500 mg DHA.

VITAMINS AND MINERALS

Vitamin C from Acerola: Vitamin C from acerola is pure and natural, unlike the usual vitamin C supplements, which are chemically synthesized. Acerola vitamin C can boost our body's immunity, prevent abnormal growth, and fight cellular aging. It is recommended that you take 500 mg per day.

Vitamin B6 and **B12**: Vitamin B6 is essential for the production of antibodies to fight infection. It also helps in maintaining the body's glucose levels. Vitamin B12 or cobalamin is needed by our body to properly process carbohydrates and fats. The best sources include grass-fed beef (in particular, beef liver), dairy, clams, salmon, and tuna. For supplements, use 2.4 mcg of B12 and 1.3 mg of B6.

Vitamin D: Vitamin D is a fat-soluble vitamin that promotes calcium absorption in the intestines. It also supports neuromuscular and immune functions throughout the body. Vitamin D is mostly found in all-natural pork, organic raw milk, cod liver oil, swordfish, organic egg yolks, tuna, and salmon. Use 500 IUs or 5 mcg per day if using a supplement.

Vitamin A: Aside from the fact that it is good for our eyes, vitamin A, or retinol, functions as an important hormone-like growth factor called retinoic acid, supporting the body's epithelial cells. Vitamin A is best found in dark leafy vegetables like spinach and kale. Organic egg yolks can also be a good source of vitamin A. If using a supplement, 900 mcg per day is the recommended dosage.

Calcium: The main function of this mineral is to help our body maintain strong bones. It is also vital for proper muscle function and nerve transmission. Calcium is best found in organic raw dairy products like milk and cheese. If using a supplement, take 1000 mg per day.

Salt: Salt is an essential nutrient to all living things. Necessary to regulate the water content of our body, salt is best when it is natural and pure. Refined table salt is bad for health, as it is processed and stripped of key minerals and nutrients. Without the right type of salt, the body can become prone to many kinds of health problems and diseases like high blood pressure, respiratory problems, accelerated aging, cellular degeneration, blood sugar problems, kidney diseases, liver failure, adrenal exhaustion, and even heart attacks. By consuming table salt, you are actually depriving your body of the natural and healthy minerals it needs.

Table Salt: This is the most commonly known salt, used by most people for cooking, baking, and food preservation. Table salt is refined and processed. It lacks 82 out of the 84 essential minerals found in salt. Left behind there is only sodium and chloride.

Celtic Sea Salt: Iodine, calcium, magnesium, iron, manganese, zinc, and potassium are some of the live minerals and trace elements that can be found in Celtic sea salt. Celtic sea salt supplies our body with the vital 84 trace minerals. In addition, Celtic sea salt provides a balanced quantity of magnesium, which removes unused sodium quickly from the body through the kidneys before it causes any harm.

HEALING THE BODY WITH CELTIC SEA SALT

A great source of trace minerals, Celtic sea salt holds remarkable healing properties that have the exact opposite effect of table salt. One of its many benefits is that it helps nourish us with minerals that our body is deficient in. Basically, it maintains the nutrient equilibrium in our body. Celtic sea salt is also particularly important in mucus elimination. Other useful benefits of Celtic sea salt are:

- Helps in sinus and bronchial congestion: when taken before sleep, Celtic sea salt gives relief to a person with sinus and bronchial congestion because it breaks up the congested mucus. This helps the person sleep better at night.

- Regulates and maintains blood pressure: Many believe that salt causes high blood pressure, but the truth is, refined salt in many cases has only shown to raise blood pressure by 1-4 mmHg. In reality, carbohydrates are far more culpable for widespread cases of high blood pressure. Celtic sea salt on the other hand has been proven to normalize blood pressure. Like a sponge, this good salt actually searches your body for detrimental sodium deposits before removing them from your body. Only a pure and natural salt has the ability to bring your blood pressure down if it is high, and also bring it up if it is too low.[19]

- Allows you to sleep more peacefully:
- Take half a teaspoon of Celtic sea salt with warm water before going to bed and you'll have a deeper and more

restful sleep. Celtic sea salt actually promotes a longer and more refreshing sleep without causing you to wake up needing to urinate in the middle of the night.

- Treats water retention: Again, contrary to popular belief, pure and natural salt does not cause water retention. It is actually only commercial table salt that can cause water retention. Celtic sea salt even does the opposite; it helps the body balance out the electrolyte minerals, releasing retained water in the process.

- Eliminates kidney stones: There have been reports that Celtic sea salt has the ability to dissolve kidney stones. For more information, visit: www.juicing-for-health.com/sea-salt-health-benefits.html [20]

- Potassium. A very important mineral, potassium is essential for the proper functioning of cells, organs, and tissues in the body. Bananas, coconuts, and organic potato skins are great sources of potassium. If using a supplement, 4,700 mg per day is best.

- Magnesium. Magnesium can do several things for your body, including relaxing your nerves and muscles, building and strengthening bones, and keeping your blood in proper circulation. Dark leafy greens give the right kind and amount of magnesium; 50 mg per day is the target dosage for a supplement.

- Manganese. Manganese can help keep your bones strong and healthy as well as promote the optimal function of the thyroid gland. Moreover, manganese helps your body utilize many key nutrients including thiamin and ascorbic acid. The best sources are brown rice and spelt. If using a supplement, use 2.3 mg per day.

- Zinc and Iron. Iron and zinc are two essential nutrients for our body. Iron is needed for blood production while zinc is great for our immune functions. Great sources of zinc and iron are organic grass-fed beef and raw dairy like milk and cheese. Oysters also have tremendous amounts of zinc and iron. If using a supplement, it is suggested to take 8 mg per day of iron and 11 mg per day of zinc.

- Caffeine. We know caffeine from our daily dose of coffee, tea, soda, and energy drinks. What we don't know is that too much caffeine can be toxic; that is why it is strongly recommended to limit caffeine intake to about 100 mg or less per day and ensure it comes from natural sources. It is ideal to take this amount of caffeine 30 minutes before a workout or exercise. Caffeine is a central nervous system stimulant, so it is suggested not to use or take caffeine after 4 p.m., as it will disturb your sleep cycles, affecting vital hormone production.

CREATINE AND AMINO ACIDS

Creatine can be used for strength, size, or to visibly tone and firm muscles. There are many forms of creatine, but generally, 5 to 20 grams per day and 60 minutes before exercise is the ideal intake.

L-Glutamine speeds up the recovery process by promoting cell and tissue repair. It can also help in muscle building, aiding in cell volumization, making a person appear bigger and fuller than usual. The ideal dosage is five to ten grams before and after exercise.

Branched Chain Amino Acids known for their muscle-building and antimuscle breakdown capabilities. Five to ten grams of this before and after workouts is ideal.

N-Acetyl-Tyrosine is great for energy. It is often used when a person is trying to reduce his or her consumption of caffeine. Taking 500 mg of N-Acetyl-Tyrosine one to three times per day is recommended. And unlike L-Tyrosine which stimulates both dopamine and norepinephrine production, and can make you crash, N-Acetyl-Tyrosine primarily works on the dopamine pathway which is less likely to lead to fatigue.

DLPA is a combination of two forms of the amino acid phenylalanine. DLPA is good for boosting the mood-elevating chemicals in the brain, specifically dopamine and nor-epinephrine. DLPA can specifically help fight mild depression, increase mental alertness, increase energy, and allay chronic pain. Because L-phenylalanine is a precursor to the stimulating catecholamines, D-phenylalanine (DPA) may be more effective for people who find DLPA to be excessively stimulating. The recommended dosage of DLPA is 1,000 - 1,500 mg per day.

L- trytophan & 5-HTP increase serotonin in the brain. 5-HTP is derived from tryptophan and is the immediate precursor to serotonin. These amino acids may help with weight loss because a lack of serotonin in the brain may trigger binge eating that accompanies a low mood. 5-HTP is effective for most people, but for some, L-tryptophan works better. For mild depression, 50-100 mg per day of 5-HTP is effective; while 600-900 mg per day of 5-HTP is better for appetite control. For L-tryptophan, 500-1,500 mg taken once or twice a day between meals or right before bedtime is ideal.

SUPERFOODS (BASED ON NUTRIENT AND ANTIOXIDANT DENSITY)

Nutrient Dense Superfoods: Organic whole eggs, full fat raw dairy, and meat from grass-fed cows naturally contain most of the vitamins and minerals outlined in the supplement section and are in a highly bio-available form.

Antioxidant Dense Superfoods: Antioxidant dense superfoods include the following:

Maca: a radish-like root, maca (Lepidium meyenii) is an herbaceous biennial plant locally found in Bolivia and the high Andes of Peru. Maca is commonly used as a root vegetable or medicinal herb; the root is known in indigenous Andean cultures to be nourishing and healing.

Maca can boost a person's libido, increase their stamina and energy, and also fight off fatigue. It also helps the body adapt to stress and regulates the stress factors forced upon it. There have also been studies that show four alkaloids present in Maca.

Camu: the Camu or cacari are small red berries known worldwide as one of nature's essential vitamin pills because they contain a higher dose of natural vitamin C than any other food.

Organically grown primarily in Peru, camu is carefully picked and processed to protect and maximize the efficacy and nutrient potential of this super berry. It is often used for its nutritional and medicinal qualities because of its incredibly high vitamin C content.

Camu has 30 to 60 times more vitamin C than the typical orange, making it a mega-C carrying fruit. Camu contains other equally important nutritional elements such as a wide range of antioxidants, amino acids, phytochemicals, and vitamins such as beta-carotene and the mineral potassium. It is a powerful whole food carrier of natural phytonutrients, making it superior to the usual isolated forms of man-made pills. It effectively enables the best possible consumption of nutrients within the body.

Cacao: Cacao is simply chocolate in its raw form. It has an incredibly high iron content. Moreover, cacao helps increase serotonin in the brain.

Maqui: Native to the Patagonia region of Chile, maqui berries are regularly harvested and eaten by the Mapuche Indians. Mapuche Indians are one of the longest living people in the world, leading researchers to believe there is a strong correlation between their Maqui diet and their disease-free healthy longevity. Several scientific researchers have confirmed that the protective nutrients of the Maqui berries have made the health and lives of the Mapuche Indians better.

Maqui berries have a very high oxygen radical absorbance capacity (ORAC) value, which is a way of measuring the antioxidant effects of food. Maqui berries hold more antioxidant properties than any other fruit. They also have high amounts of flavonoids like anthocyanins and polyphenols. In addition, they are an amazing source of calcium, vitamin C, potassium, and iron.

The abundant supply of health-improving phytochemicals provided by the Maqui berries will greatly enhance the nutritional benefits of other foods or recipes, even with just a small amount.

SUCCESS STRATEGIES

NUTRITIONAL GUIDELINES

So you've learned a great deal of useful information by this point, but that information is only as valuable as the way you use it. Here are the appropriate steps you can take to successfully implement the philosophies of this book into your lifestyle:

STEP 1 – NUTRITIONAL DEFICIENCY

Almost all of us have one or more nutritional deficiencies, and trying to perform a complete overhaul on your diet all at once is unlikely to stick. And because our energy levels, appetites, strengths, endurance, and moods are all dependent on getting adequate amounts of the essential nutrients, even a small deficiency will throw everything off. You could eat "clean," go on a low-carb diet, do Paleo, be vegan, or count calories and still not feel great. The only way to eradicate this problem is to identify your deficiencies from day one, and then gradually eliminate them. The most common deficiencies include water (dehydration), vitamins and minerals, protein (amino acids), and essential fatty acids. As mentioned before, do not try to attack all of these at once. The best results I've seen have come from simply going after the most important, which are your essential fats. Because 95% of the population is deficient in essential fatty acids, you can see tremendous results simply by adding three to six grams of fermented fish oil to your diet every day. Look for a brand that has 1,000 mg per capsule with 500 mg from EPA and 500 mg from DHA. After you have successfully integrated this into your diet for two weeks, then challenge yourself to your next habit milestone (e.g., drinking more water).

STEP 2 – FOOD QUANTITY AND QUALITY

After addressing the micronutrients, you can move on to the macronutrients. As you already know, I'm not an advocate of counting calories – it just doesn't work long-term. In addition, counting calories is really just a crutch for a weak mind-gut connection, a connection that must be repaired to achieve natural hunger and appetite suppression. Not to mention that calorie counting can be off by as much as 25% because of things like incorrect labeling and laboratory errors. So how can you possibly control consumption without counting calories? Here's how: use your hand as a yardstick for each meal.

For Men:

- 1-2 palms of protein-dense foods
- 1-2 fists of vegetables
- 1-2 cupped handfuls of carbohydrate-dense foods
- 1-2 thumbs of fat-dense foods

For Women:

- 1 palm of protein-dense foods
- 1 fist of vegetables
- 1 cupped handful of carbohydrate-dense foods
- 1 thumb of fat-dense foods

You can adjust your portion sizes up or down to match your body type and goals. For example, for muscle gain, have two palms of protein-dense foods at every meal and another thumb of fat or handful of carbs. For fat loss, have only one palm of protein, one thumb of fat, and one cupped handful of carbs, eaten slowly (to ensure you only eat until 80% full).

For most people, eliminating nutrient deficiencies and consuming the correct quality and portion size of food will make all the difference. But for those who have more advanced goals or perhaps are already doing the above, focus on food composition. The simplest way to do this is to break it down by body type.

The following is a list of common body types:

Ectomorph (naturally skinny)

Mesomorph (naturally muscular)

Endomorph (naturally heavier)

Here are examples of these:

Ectomorphs

Let's begin with ectomorphs. They are thin, have smaller bone structures and thinner limbs, and are generally endurance athletes (or at least look that way). They tend to either have a high output from their sympathetic nervous system and/or thyroid, or are more sensitive to epinephrine and norepinephrine (catecholamines). Essentially, they have fast metabolisms. Because of these traits, ectomorphs tend to tolerate carbs well, so a higher carbohydrate diet (with moderate protein and lower fat intake) for this body type generally works best. Somewhere around 55% carbs, 30% protein, and 15% fat would be ideal here.

This is what that would look like:

For Men:

- 2 palms of protein-dense foods
- 2 fists of vegetables
- 3 cupped handfuls of carb-dense foods
- 1 thumb of fat-dense foods

For Women:

- 1 palm of protein-dense foods
- 1 fist of vegetables
- 2 cupped handfuls of carb-dense foods
- 1/2 thumb of fat-dense foods

Mesomorphs

Mesomorphs typically have an athletic build, medium-sized bone structure, and a fair amount of lean mass if they exercise regularly. For mesomorphs, excess calories usually go to building lean mass and dense bones. They also tend to have more growth hormone and testosterone, and thus can usually gain muscle and stay lean easily. This body type does best with a balanced diet of approximately 40% carbs, 30% protein, and 30% fat.

Here's what that might look like:

For Men:

- 2 palms of protein-dense foods
- 2 fists of vegetables
- 2 cupped handfuls of carb-dense foods
- 2 thumbs of fat dense foods

For Women:

- 1 palm of protein-dense foods
- 1 fist of vegetables
- 1 cupped handful of carb-dense foods
- 1 thumb of fat-dense foods

Endomorphs

Endomorphs have higher fat mass and total body mass. They have larger bone structures, stronger parasympathetic nervous systems (designed for comfort, not speed), and slower metabolic rates. As a result, they are naturally less active, store excess calories as body fat more easily, and do not tolerate carbohydrates well. Therefore, a diet comprised of 25% carbs, 35% protein, and 40% fat will work best for this body type. (Do not get hung up on the math here, remember you are going to measure everything using your own hand.)

Here's what that might look like:

For Men:

- 2 palms of protein-dense foods
- 2 fists of vegetables
- 1 cupped handful of carb-dense foods
- 3 thumbs of fat-dense foods

For Women:

- 1 palm of protein-dense foods
- 1 fist of vegetables
- 1/2 cupped handful of carb-dense foods
- 2 thumbs of fat-dense foods

EXAMPLES OF CARB, FAT, AND PROTEIN SOURCES:

Carbs:

brown rice, sprouted grain bread, sweet potatoes, quinoa

Fat:

raw butter, raw whole milk, cold-pressed olive oil, coconut oil

Protein:

wild-caught fish, free-range omega-3 eggs, grass-fed beef, organic chicken, New Zealand lamb

ESTIMATING YOUR NEEDS

BODY TYPE & GENERAL GOAL:

BODY TYPE	GENERAL GOAL	CARBS	PROTEIN	FAT
Ectomorphic	Muscle Gain	55%	30%	15%
Mesomorphic	Muscle Gain/ Body Fat Loss	40%	30%	30%
Endomorphic	Fat Loss	25%	35%	40%

STEP 3 – FINE TUNING

Now that we've addressed the requisites, we can progress to fine-tuning your diet. The most important thing to keep in mind here is that none of the following should be integrated until all of the above have been consistently addressed (i.e., removing deficiencies, controlling calorie intake, eating for your body type).

MEAL TIMING

I, and probably everyone else, used to think that eating small, frequent meals throughout the day was the best way to keep your metabolism high and appetite low. But studies proved otherwise and suggest that simply eating the right foods in the right amounts is enough. This means that meal timing is secondary and can be left to your personal preference. The key here is to listen to your own body and adapt the strategy that works best for you (e.g., eating small meals frequently vs. a few big meals infrequently).[21]

ADAPTING BASED ON BLOOD TYPE

The Blood Type Diet, created by naturopath Peter J. D'Adamo, offers more specificity when it comes to individualizing your diet. If the guidelines for your blood type are incongruous with your body type, your blood type should take precedence because it is unique:

Type O blood: these people function best on higher-protein diets rich in lean meat, poultry, fish, and vegetables, and light on grains, beans, and dairy.

Type A blood: this blood type will feel best on a diet lower in meat and higher in fruits and vegetables, beans and legumes, and whole grains.

TYPE B BLOOD: This type should avoid corn, wheat, buckwheat, lentils, tomatoes, peanuts, and sesame seeds. They do best with green vegetables, eggs, meats, and raw dairy.

TYPE AB BLOOD: This type does best with seafood, dairy, and green vegetables. Type ABs often have low stomach acid, so it is necessary for them to avoid caffeine, alcohol, and smoked or cured meats.[22]

CARB CYCLING

Carbohydrate cycling is a great way to fine tune for fat loss, lean muscle gain, and even just getting in shape. What it implies is that you will eat more carbohydrates on the days you exercise at a high-volume or high-intensity, and fewer carbohydrates on low-intensity, low-volume workout days or on rest days. The focus is on carbohydrates and not fats or proteins because carbs tend to have the greatest effect on body composition and how you look and feel. Because cycling carbohydrates will also cycle calories, it will help keep your metabolism in high gear at all times, without the adverse effects of long-term calorie/carb restriction.

Here's how to do it for fat loss:

On weight lifting days or workout days involving high-volume or high-intensity exercise, add more starchy carbs to your diet.

On non-lifting days or workout days involving low-volume or low-intensity exercise, eat a diet comprised of mainly protein, vegetables, and fats. Limit carbohydrate intake.

For more significant fat loss, try this eating schedule:

> Day 1 - Low Calorie & Low Carb
>
> Day 2 - Low Calorie & Low Carb
>
> Day 3 - High Calorie & Low Carb
>
> Day 4 - Average Calorie & Average Carb
>
> Day 5 - Low Calorie & Low Carb
>
> Day 6 - Low Calorie & Low Carb
>
> Day 7 - High Calorie & High Carb

Here's how to do it for lean muscle gain and to optimize your muscle to fat ratio:

> Day 1 - eat 20% fewer carbs than usual - basically omitting carbs from one of your typical meals.
>
> Day 2 - average carbohydrate consumption
>
> Day 3 - eat 20% more carbs than usual - basically, adding carbs to one of your typically lower carb meals.
>
> Repeat days 1-3

For athletes, higher carbohydrate diets can aid performance. Here's how you can use carb cycling to your athletic advantage:

During training periods - consume 55% carbs, 25% protein, and 20% fat daily.

Three to four days prior to competition – consume 70% carbs, 15% protein, and 15% fat daily.[23]

INTERMITTENT FASTING

Traditional intermittent fasting (IF) entails going twelve to sixteen hours without eating anything. This can be effective for weight loss but wreaks havoc on fat loss and muscle tone. Another more recently popular craze is the use of medium-chain fats and coffee to augment the IF. To perform IF with coffee, here's what you would do:

Do not consume food past 8 p.m. the night before you begin your fast.

Upon waking, drink two cups of organic coffee blended with 1-2 Tbsp of Kerrygold butter and 1-2 Tbsp of MCT or coconut oil.

Continue drinking this coffee blend, as desired, until 2 p.m. (do not drink the coffee past this time or you will disrupt your sleep cycles).

From 2 p.m. – 8 p.m. you "feast" (the number of meals and calorie count is irrelevant). If fasting for eighteen hours is too challenging for you, start with a shorter fast and increase incrementally.

The Mechanisms Behind Intermittent Fasting with MCTs & Coffee

Reason #1: mTOR

mTOR stands for "Mammalian Target of Rapamycin." mTOR is a major mechanism that increases protein synthesis in your muscles. Both exercise and coffee raise cellular energy use while simultaneously inhibiting your muscle building mechanisms for a brief period, which causes it to spike and build even more muscle as soon as you eat. There are three primary ways to raise mTOR: intermittent fasting, exercise, and coffee.

Fasting with MCTs satisfies all three ways to inhibit mTOR, causing a bigger rebound and better use of your food for muscle building. Plain intermittent fasting doesn't use coffee, so it only hits one, or possibly two of the three possible mTOR triggers. This style of fasting works better because it can use all three mechanisms. The beauty is that an all-fat breakfast doesn't make your body think it's broken the fast, so you get the benefits of traditional intermittent fasting without the same deprivation, hunger pangs, sluggishness, brain fog, or any of the other generally poor mood-associated symptoms.

Reason #2: Ketosis

Traditional intermittent fasting helps you enter ketosis (a fat-burning "mode") but this ends once you eat carb-containing foods at the end of the fast. By using MCT oil in your coffee, you increase the rate at which you go into ketosis, so it not only fuels your brain but also helps you stay in ketosis, even in the presence of some carbs in your diet.

Reason #3: Increased Metabolism

Unlike traditional intermittent fasting, this style fast increases your metabolism by up to 20 percent.[24]

Be Cautious About Intermittent Fasting

Although some experts have recently hailed intermittent fasting as almost a gold standard approach to weight loss, it isn't for everyone and can often make your metabolism crash.

Besides being painful and risking cognitive deficits on the days you fast, the ability to lose weight this way is likely not a good long-term solution. People who believe this will help them lose weight maintain that fasting tricks the body into going into a fat-burning state. This means the body will burn stored fat when faced with low-calorie consumption. What really happens is that the body continues to store the fat while it tends to burn lean tissue. This means that fasting actually has the opposite effect of what you are looking for. It turns out that the body actually responds to fasting by storing more energy in the form of fat.

The question then becomes: how about the stories of people fasting and successfully losing weight? People who research fasting claim that, on the days when people fast, they tend to eat a lot of fruits and vegetables because they are low in calories. This substitution of nutrient-dense for calorie-dense food, plus a lowering of sodium intake, which results in less water retention, helps the faster lose a little bit of weight. But this weight loss comes in the form of loss from lean muscle tissue and not from fat.

Also, fasting may help a person get in touch with their natural sense of hunger. When you fast, you feel hunger pangs that you wouldn't ordinarily feel when you eat normally. This sensitizes you to the feeling of hunger in a general way. When a person becomes more aware of true hunger, they become less sensitive to the emotional and social cues that can stimulate eating.

Even with these theorized advantages, there is little research to support the claims of fasting for weight loss. The little evidence that the diet relies upon is based on studies that lacked a randomized population and control groups. In fact, not one randomized controlled trial has been published to date according to *The American Journal of Clinical Nutrition*.

Another claim is that fasting is healthy in general. It is impossible to reduce your calorie intake to 500 calories a day without risking your body's ability to function normally. You need to be able to acquire enough dietary fat for cell membrane integrity and enough glucose for brain function. Most people require a minimum of 1,200 calories to keep up with all the vital processes the body performs.

Even when people faithfully adhere to a fasting diet, it has been shown to be no more effective for weight loss than merely restricting caloric intake. Plus, a person's appetite will increase because of the fasting, likely leading to an unrestricted feast during their feeding windows.

DANGERS OF FASTING

Intermittent fasting diets may encourage regular physical activity on the fasting days. Keeping up with regular activity despite the lowered calorie intake may put you at risk for low blood sugar, dehydration, injury, and compromised immune function.

Fasting can also be dangerous for certain subpopulations. These include women, people with type 1 diabetes, those with a history of disordered eating, and people who take prescription medication.

Sometimes, fasting is beneficial for certain medical conditions. However, this kind of fasting needs to be closely monitored by a physician. Despite the fact that intermittent fasting is popular with the public, it has yet to be demonstrated that it is safe and effective.

Instead of fasting, a wise dieting choice is to reduce your calorie intake but get a balanced diet at the same time. Also, our body gets the best benefit from fasting when we are sleeping. So try and develop a "kitchen closed" rule where you take your last bite of food about two hours before bedtime. This is important for two reasons. First, you are inactive in the later evening. This means you will likely not immediately burn off the calories you consume then. And second, you may feel more refreshed and alert the next morning. This is because your body didn't have to overwork itself by digesting the snack overnight.

For many people, a ketogenic or Paleo style diet will wreck their metabolism. Instead, I recommend a Weston A. Price style diet. This type of diet consists of eating primarily pasture raised sources of animal fats and proteins (i.e. grass fed butter, raw whole milk, pasture raised eggs, grass fed beef, duck fat, etc.). The diet isn't all carnivorous though, it integrates many plants and natural carbohydrates.

To give you a little background on Weston A. Price, he was a dentist by trade who traveled the world studying traditional diets. What he discovered was astounding. Many indigenous peoples, without access to modern technology or dentistry, had perfectly straight teeth, no wisdom teeth that needed to be pulled, no heart disease, and virtually optimal health. The diets he studied varied, of course, based on what foods each group had access to, but here were the common denominators:

- Their diets were high in animal-based Vitamins A & D (such as cod liver oil)
- They ate large amounts of animal products, and none were vegetarian or vegan
- They did not consume refined carbohydrates or packaged goods – they only ate REAL FOOD

What was most interesting about Weston's findings was the way he applied them to treating his dental patients. He realized his patients were missing the critical nutrients that were so high in these foods, and this deficiency in their diets was leading to tooth decay as well as health decay. He also realized they didn't actually have to completely change their current diets. Instead, he found he could achieve results by having his patients integrate the following into their daily diets on top of what they were already eating:

- 3/4 tsp cod liver oil and butter oil in a small amount of orange juice
- A stew with green vegetables, carrots, meat, and bone marrow. These would be rotated with organ meats and fish chowder.
- Fruit, that has been slightly cooked
- Rolls made from freshly ground wheat with natural butter
- Two glasses of whole raw milk

After eating all of the above, in addition to whatever else they wanted, they were allowed to go back for seconds or thirds if they were still hungry. Most impressively, with these diet additions he was able to reverse tooth decay without any oral surgery as well as help some of them lose weight and optimize their health.

The style of eating may be most useful for weight loss as well as helping reduce inflammation, prevent blood sugar volatility and cravings, improve gut health, dental health, and longevity.

WORKOUT NUTRITION

Everyone always wants to know how to time meals properly for workouts, and what to have right before, during, and after a workout.

The answer is simple: unless you are an elite athlete (in which case eating an appropriate meal two hours before would be relevant) it does not matter. And by elite athlete I am referring to someone who is training specifically for maximal muscle adaptation and training with high volume and intensity, potentially multiple times per day.

Besides eating a proper meal two hours before, for elite athletes I recommend a low-calorie, low-carb BCAA (branched-chain amino acid) drink or a protein plus carbohydrate drink during and/or after workouts for optimal recovery.

For everyone else, I recommend that you eat normally around your workout, and simply sip on five to fifteen grams of BCAAs mixed in one liter of water during your workout.[25]

7 CRITICAL SUCCESS HABITS

1. Eat a serving of **vegetables** with every meal. Vegetables are packed with minerals, vitamins, enzymes, and fiber – all necessary to regulate your digestion, stabilize blood sugar, and increase alkalinity (counteracting blood acidity). Also, because protein and grains increase the acidity of the blood (zapping your energy, bone density, and muscle mass), it is vital that you consume enough vegetables to balance this.

2. Consume **healthy fats** every day. Good saturated fats and monounsaturated fats (MUFAs) should be a regular part of your daily diet. Aim to get a third of your healthy fat intake from each. This will help improve your body composition, mental clarity, and overall fitness. You can get more saturated fat from animal products (e.g., raw whole milk or grass-fed beef) and coconut or palm oil, MUFAs from things like extra virgin olive oil and avocado, as well as fermented cod liver oil supplements.

3. Eat **real food** over meal replacements when possible. Grab a bar or shake only when it's absolutely necessary. It's understandable that when you're pressed for time you need a quick substitute for a real meal. But even the best meal replacements are no comparison to the vitamin, mineral, enzyme, and phytochemical power of whole foods.

4. Eat to **80% full** at each meal. Overeating is a common problem for most Americans. Even if your goal isn't fat loss, eating to 80% full ensures you aren't distressing your body's natural hunger signals and mechanisms.

5. Eat as wide a **variety** of good food as you can. It is advantageous for our health and vigor to acquire our nutrition from a variety of seasonal foods and sources. We are all culpable of being creatures of habit, but you have to break out of your comfort zone and expose your body to a breadth of foods to maximize your immunity, energy, and body composition.

6. Create a **weekly meal plan**. Planning out your meals for the week is a best practice you cannot overlook. As the saying goes, if you fail to plan, you plan to fail. Later in the book, you'll see a sample eating plan with a corresponding grocery list to set you up for success.

7. Avoid **drinking your calories**. Unless you're blending your own shakes from whole foods or consuming an exercise recovery drink comprised of coconut water, amino acids, and optional creatine, you should avoid most other calorie-containing beverages. Avoid the obvious sodas (and diet sodas) but also be wary of concentrated juices. The majority of these drinks, like most carbohydrate-rich beverages, are high in added sugar as well as preservatives and other artificial ingredients – all a detriment to your fat metabolism and energy levels.

TAKING ACTION

17 POWER FOODS

Track your power food consumption and aim for FIVE OF EACH POWER FOOD PER WEEK.

We suggest you make copies of the chart (on the following page), put it on your fridge, and check off your progress throughout the week to ensure you get in all of your power foods.

	1	2	3	4	5
Grass-Fed Red Meats					
Wild-Caught Fish					
Omega-3, Free-Range Eggs					
Skim or Whole Raw Milk					
Quinoa					
Raw Cacao					
Spinach					
Kale					
Cruciferous Vegetables					
Sprouted Grains					
Avocado					
Walnuts, Almonds (raw and soaked), or Pistachios					
Fermented Fish Oil					
Free-Range Chicken or Turkey					
Flax Seeds/Oil					
Coconut or Palm Oil					
Extra Virgin Olive Oil, Cold-Pressed					

IMPLEMENTATION SCHEDULE

Over the next twelve weeks, we are going to help you change your habits so you can more easily transition our dietary philosophy into your lifestyle.

The first six weeks are focused on including new habits into your lifestyle (so don't change your other dietary habits just yet), while weeks seven through twelve attempt to begin eliminating poor nutritional choices.

Week 1-6

Select one of the following new daily habits to include in your diet each week:

- Drink one cup of raw whole milk
- Drink one cup of water with half a lemon upon waking
- Consume fruits and vegetables regularly (sign up for a CSA to obtain local organic fruits and vegetables)
- Consume three to six grams of fermented cod liver oil
- Consume three servings of fermented foods (e.g., kombucha tea, natural sauerkraut, kefir)
- Supplement with a probiotic daily

Week 7-9

Select one of the following new habit changes to commit to completely each week:

- Eliminate caffeine consumption
- Eliminate alcohol consumption
- Eliminate artificial sweeteners

Week 10-12

Select two of the following new habit changes to commit to completely each week:

- Eliminate gluten consumption
- Eliminate pesticide consumption
- Eliminate toxic substances such as carrageenan (i.e. almond milk, coconut milk, etc.) and goitrogenic toxins (like those found in unsoaked almonds)
- Eliminate soy from diet
- Eliminate refined sugar from diet
- Eliminate all processed foods (including processed carbohydrates and oils)

CONCLUSION

Our hope is that the principles of this book become second nature to you – that the information contained here helps you live a happier, healthier, and longer life.

This book was written to inspire and educate people like you who are ready to change their lives for the better.

Bear in mind that knowledge must be supported by action if anything is to be achieved. If you are cognizant of your eating habits and emotional ties with food and you take action to change these habits, victory will follow.

With little time and effort, the ideas in this book should empower you to face and overcome all the obstacles you may encounter regarding your health.

We are constantly barraged by new fad diets, nutritional trends, and other fitness tricks that promise instant success. Most people try these fad diets to slim down or lose weight, and in some cases are successful. The catch, of course, is that they lose weight at the expense of their overall health. Any fad diet promising rapid, dramatic fat loss is likely to deprive the body of vital nutrients. Inevitably, these diets are extremely difficult to maintain, leading to the eventual rebound in weight gain. It is best not to let society dictate your health. In a world where misinformation is increasingly pervasive, you can only rely on the facts delivered by the passionate, less-greedy sorts. Your local CSAs and farms are a good place to start, and some commercial health food markets are acceptable as well.

If you want to learn more or have a question in mind, we offer 24/7 support via live chat or text message at Exerscribe.com.

Think clearly. Live healthy. Good luck in your quest to greatness.

Thomas Jefferson once said, "In matters of style, swim with the current. In matters of principle, stand like a rock."

28 Day Meal Plan + Shopping List

Initial Shopping List

Non-perishables (and Extended Expirations) FOR 28 DAYS:

Peanut Butter

Brown Rice

Quinoa

Extra Virgin Olive Oil

Olive Oil Non-Stick Spray

Worcestershire Sauce

Teriyaki Sauce

Apple Cider Vinegar

Balsamic Vinegar

Butter

Salt

Pepper

Dried Basil

Ground Oregano

Turmeric

Chili Powder

Cinnamon

Vanilla Extract

Red Curry Paste

Sriracha

Ketchup

Gluten-Free Bread Crumbs

Brown Rice Flour

WEEK 1 MEAL PLAN

Day 1

Pre-Breakfast	1 Glass Lemon Water/Supplements
Breakfast	Apple, Grapefruit, and Spinach Smoothie, Eggs
Snack	1 Glass Kombucha, Celery and Peanut Butter
Lunch	Cobb Sandwich, Carrot Sticks
Snack	1 Glass Raw Whole Milk
Dinner	No Carb Lasagna

Day 2

Pre-Breakfast	1 Glass Lemon Water/Supplements
Breakfast	Eggs & Sprouted Grain Toast w/Peanut Butter
Snack	Sliced Avocado w/Salt, Pepper, and Lime
Lunch	No Carb Lasagna Leftovers
Snack	Celery & Peanut Butter
Dinner	Sausage-Stuffed Peppers

Day 3

Pre-Breakfast	1 Glass Lemon Water/Supplements
Breakfast	Apple, Grapefruit, and Spinach Smoothie, Eggs
Snack	Raw Cheddar Cheese, Carrot Sticks
Lunch	Sausage-Stuffed Peppers Leftovers
Snack	1 Glass Raw Kefir, Carrot Sticks
Dinner	Peanut Butter Chicken, Side Salad w/Olive Oil and Lemon Juice Dressing

Day 4

Pre-Breakfast	1 Glass Lemon Water/Supplements
Breakfast	Eggs & Sprouted Grain Toast w/Peanut Butter
Snack	Sliced Avocado w/Salt, Pepper, and Lime
Lunch	Peanut Butter Chicken Leftovers
Snack	1 Glass Raw Whole Milk, 1 Apple
Dinner	Stuffed Butternut Squash

Day 5

Pre-Breakfast	1 Glass Lemon Water/Supplements
Breakfast	Apple, Grapefruit, and Spinach Smoothie, Eggs
Snack	1 Glass Kombucha, Celery and Peanut Butter
Lunch	Stuffed Butternut Squash Leftovers
Snack	1 Glass raw Kefir, Carrot Sticks
Dinner	Spinach & Goat Cheese Chicken Burgers, Easy Cucumber Salad

Day 6

Pre-Breakfast	1 Glass Lemon Water/Supplements
Breakfast	Eggs & Sprouted Grain Toast w/Peanut Butter
Snack	Raw Cheddar Cheese, Carrot Sticks
Lunch	Spinach & Goat Cheese Chicken Burgers Leftovers w/Easy Cucumber Salad
Snack	Celery and Peanut Butter
Dinner	Teriyaki Chicken Bowl, Side Salad w/Olive Oil and Lemon Juice Dressing

Day 7

Pre-Breakfast	1 Glass Lemon Water/Supplements
Breakfast	Coconut Milk Breakfast Quinoa w/Toasted Coconut and Berries
Snack	1 Glass Kombucha, Raw Cheddar Cheese
Lunch	Teriyaki Chicken Bowl Leftovers
Snack	1 Glass Raw Whole Milk, 1 Apple
Dinner	Avocado Chicken Salad, Sprouted Grain Toast

WEEK 1 SHOPPING LIST

(Weekly staples are listed in all CAPS)

KOMBUCHA

LEMONS

SPINACH

CELERY

CARROTS

EGGS

CHÈVRE GOAT CHEESE

GOAT or RAW
CHEDDAR CHEESE

GLUTEN-FREE or
SPROUTED GRAIN
BREAD

GREEK or GOAT
YOGURT (PLAIN)

RAW WHOLE MILK

Kefir

Apples

Grapefruit

Avocado

Tomatoes

Blueberries

)

Red, Green, & Yellow Bell
Peppers

Kale

Butternut Squash

Cucumber

Mushrooms

Limes

Fresh Parsley

Mixed Greens for Salad

Bacon

Shredded Coconut

Canned Coconut Milk

Canned Crushed Tomatoes

Canned Diced Tomatoes

Chicken Thighs

Ground Chicken

Chicken Sausage

GF or Sprouted Grain
Hamburger Buns (or Use
Sliced Bread

WEEK 2 MEAL PLAN

Day 1

Pre-Breakfast	1 Glass Lemon Water/Supplements
Breakfast	1 Glass Raw Whole Milk, Sprouted Grain Toast w/Butter or Peanut Butter, 1/2 Orange
Snack	1 Glass Kombucha, Carrot Sticks
Lunch	Avocado Chicken Salad Leftovers
Snack	Spinach Artichoke Dip w/Celery
Dinner	Bacon Lentil Soup

Day 2

Pre-Breakfast	1 Glass Lemon Water/Supplements
Breakfast	Banana, Orange, and Spinach Smoothie, Eggs
Snack	1 Glass Kombucha, 1/4 Cup Cashews
Lunch	Bacon Lentil Soup Leftovers, 1 Pear
Snack	Spinach Artichoke Dip w/ Celery
Dinner	Spaghetti Squash w/Turkey Meatballs, Side Salad w/Olive Oil and Lemon Juice Dressing

Day 3

Pre-Breakfast	1 Glass Lemon Water/Supplements
Breakfast	1 Glass Raw Whole Milk & Sprouted Grain Toast w/Butter or Peanut Butter, 1/2 Orange
Snack	Greek or Goat Yogurt w/Pear Slices
Lunch	Spaghetti Squash Leftovers
Snack	Spinach Artichoke Dip w/ Celery
Dinner	Pork Ribs, Balsamic Roasted Artichokes

Day 4

Pre-Breakfast	1 Glass Lemon Water/Supplements
Breakfast	Banana, Orange, and Spinach Smoothie, Eggs
Snack	1 Glass Kombucha, 1/4 Cup Cashews
Lunch	Pork Ribs Leftovers, Side Salad w/Olive Oil and Lemon Juice Dressing
Snack	1 Glass Raw Whole Milk, Carrot Sticks
Dinner	Yogurt Broiled Halibut, Creamed Kale Stuffed Sweet Potatoes

Day 5

Pre-Breakfast	1 Glass Lemon Water/Supplements
Breakfast	1 Glass Raw Whole Milk & Sprouted Grain Toast w/Butter or Peanut Butter, 1/2 Orange
Snack	Raw Cheddar Cheese, Carrot Sticks
Lunch	Yogurt Broiled Halibut, Creamed Kale Stuffed Sweet Potatoes Leftovers
Snack	Celery and Peanut Butter
Dinner	Turmeric Chicken, Side Salad w/Olive Oil and Lemon Juice Dressing

Day 6

Pre-Breakfast	1 Glass Lemon Water/Supplements
Breakfast	Banana, Orange, and Spinach Smoothie, Eggs
Snack	1 Glass Kombucha, 1/4 Cup Cashews
Lunch	Turmeric Chicken and Side Salad Leftovers
Snack	1 Glass Raw Whole Milk, Carrot Sticks
Dinner	Cauliflower Pizza

Day 7

Pre-Breakfast	1 Glass Lemon Water/Supplements
Breakfast	Butternut Squash Frittata
Snack	Greek or Goat Yogurt w/Pear Slices
Lunch	Cauliflower Pizza Leftovers
Snack	Celery and Peanut Butter
Dinner	Grilled Portobello Burgers

WEEK 2 SHOPPING LIST

KOMBUCHA

LEMONS

SPINACH

CELERY

CARROTS

EGGS

CHÈVRE GOAT CHEESE

GOAT or RAW
  CHEDDAR CHEESE

GLUTEN-FREE or
  SPROUTED GRAIN
  BREAD

GREEK or GOAT
  YOGURT (PLAIN)

RAW WHOLE MILK

Oranges

Bananas

Pears

Red Bell Pepper

Kale

Mushrooms

Onion

Green Onions

Spaghetti Squash

Butternut Squash

Artichokes

Sweet Potatoes

Cauliflower

Tomatoes

Portobello Mushrooms

Avocado

Mixed Greens for Salad

Chicken Legs

Sausage Links

Ground Turkey

Bacon

Pork Ribs

Halibut

Frozen Chopped Spinach

Canned Artichokes

Canned Diced Tomatoes

Cashews

Marinara Sauce

Low Sodium Chicken Broth

Fresh Rosemary

GF or Sprouted Grain
  Hamburger Buns (or use
  Sliced Bread)

Lentils

WEEK 3 MEAL PLAN

Day 1

Pre-Breakfast	1 Glass Lemon Water/Supplements
Breakfast	White Peach and Carrot Smoothie, Eggs
Snack	1 Glass Kombucha, 1/4 Cup Almonds
Lunch	Grilled Portobello Burger Leftovers
Snack	Sliced Avocado Sprinkled w/Salt, Pepper, and Lime
Dinner	Basil Pesto Pasta w/Grilled Chicken

Day 2

Pre-Breakfast	1 Glass Lemon Water/Supplements
Breakfast	Eggs, Bacon, and Sautéed Spinach
Snack	1 Glass Raw Whole Milk, Carrot Sticks
Lunch	Basil Pesto Pasta w/Grilled Chicken Leftovers
Snack	1 Glass Kombucha, 1 Apple
Dinner	Vegetable and Wild Rice Soup, Sprouted Grain Toast

Day 3

Pre-Breakfast	1 Glass Lemon Water/Supplements
Breakfast	White Peach and Carrot Smoothie, Eggs
Snack	1 Glass Kombucha, 1/4 Cup Almonds
Lunch	Wild Rice Chicken Soup Leftovers, 1 Apple
Snack	1 Glass Raw Milk, Celery and Peanut Butter
Dinner	Enchiladas w/ Tangy Avocado Cream Sauce, Side Salad w/ Olive Oil and Lemon Juice Dressing

Day 4

Pre-Breakfast	1 Glass Lemon Water/Supplements
Breakfast	Eggs, Bacon, and Sautéed Spinach
Snack	1 Glass Raw Whole Milk, Carrot Sticks
Lunch	Enchiladas w/Tangy Avocado Cream Sauce Leftovers
Snack	1 Glass Kombucha, 1 Apple
Dinner	Quinoa Coconut Chicken, Sautéed Green Beans

Day 5

Pre-Breakfast	1 Glass Lemon Water/Supplements
Breakfast	White Peach and Carrot Smoothie, Eggs
Snack	1 Glass Kombucha, 1/4 Cup Almonds
Lunch	Quinoa Coconut Chicken Leftovers, 1 Apple
Snack	Sliced Avocado Sprinkled w/Salt, Pepper, and Lime
Dinner	Italian Breaded Baked Cod, Side Salad w/Olive Oil and Lemon Juice Dressing

Day 6

Pre-Breakfast	1 Glass Lemon Water/Supplements
Breakfast	Eggs, Bacon, and Sautéed Spinach
Snack	1 Glass Raw Whole Milk, Carrot Sticks
Lunch	Italian Breaded Baked Cod and Side Salad Leftovers
Snack	1 Glass Kombucha, 1 Apple
Dinner	Cauliflower Mac n' Cheese, Sautéed Green Beans

Day 7

Pre-Breakfast	1 Glass Lemon Water/Supplements
Breakfast	Mexican Breakfast Eggs
Snack	1 Glass Kombucha, 1/4 Cup Almonds
Lunch	Cauliflower Mac n' Cheese and Sautéed Green Beans Leftovers
Snack	1 Glass Raw Milk, Celery and Peanut Butter
Dinner	Balsamic Chicken and Tomatoes, Side Salad w/Olive Oil and Lemon Juice Dressing

WEEK 3 SHOPPING LIST

KOMBUCHA

LEMONS

SPINACH

CELERY

CARROTS

EGGS

CHÈVRE GOAT CHEESE

GOAT or RAW
  CHEDDAR CHEESE

GLUTEN-FREE or
  SPROUTED GRAIN
  BREAD

GREEK or GOAT
  YOGURT (PLAIN)

RAW WHOLE MILK

White Peaches (OK Frozen
  if Fresh is Not Available)

Blueberries (OK Frozen if
  Fresh is Not Available)

Avocado

Limes

Apples

Onions

Mushrooms

Red Bell Pepper

Mixed Greens for Salad

Cauliflower

Green Beans

Cherry Tomatoes

Fresh Ginger

Fresh Basil

Chicken Legs

Chicken Thighs

Cod

Bacon

Vanilla Greek Yogurt

Almonds

Pine Nuts

Wild Rice

GF Pasta

Brown Rice Tortillas

Low-Sodium Chicken Broth

Canned Low-Sodium Refried
  Beans

Canned Low-Sodium Black
  Beans

Canned Diced Tomatoes

Canned Diced Green Chiles

Canned Enchilada Sauce

Canned Coconut Milk

WEEK 4 MEAL PLAN

Day 1

Pre-Breakfast	1 Glass Lemon Water/Supplements
Breakfast	Eggs & Sautéed Sweet Potatoes
Snack	Apple, Raw Cheddar Cheese
Lunch	Balsamic Chicken and Tomatoes Leftovers
Snack	1 Glass Kombucha, Celery and Peanut Butter
Dinner	Cheese and Broccoli Soup

Day 2

Pre-Breakfast	1 Glass Lemon Water/Supplements
Breakfast	Creamy Green Smoothie, Eggs
Snack	1 Glass Raw Milk, Celery and Peanut Butter
Lunch	Cheese and Broccoli Soup Leftovers
Snack	1 Glass Kombucha, 1 Apple
Dinner	Chicken Fried Rice, Side Salad w/Olive Oil and Lemon Juice Dressing

Day 3

Pre-Breakfast	1 Glass Lemon Water/Supplements
Breakfast	Eggs, Sprouted Grain Toast, 1/2 Orange
Snack	1 Glass Kombucha, 1/4 Cup Pistachios
Lunch	Chicken Fried Rice Leftovers
Snack	1 Glass Raw Milk, Celery and Peanut Butter
Dinner	Cilantro Lime Chicken Tacos

Day 4

Pre-Breakfast	1 Glass Lemon Water/Supplements
Breakfast	Eggs & Sautéed Sweet Potatoes
Snack	Apple, Raw Cheddar Cheese
Lunch	Cilantro Lime Chicken Tacos Leftovers
Snack	1 Glass Kombucha, Celery and Peanut Butter
Dinner	Grilled Salmon and Quinoa Spinach Salad

Day 5

Pre-Breakfast	1 Glass Lemon Water/Supplements
Breakfast	Creamy Green Smoothie, Eggs
Snack	1 Glass Raw Milk, Celery and Peanut Butter
Lunch	Grilled Salmon and Quinoa Spinach Salad Leftovers
Snack	1 Glass Kombucha, 1/4 Cup Pistachios
Dinner	Beef and Broccoli

Day 6

Pre-Breakfast	1 Glass Lemon Water/Supplements
Breakfast	Eggs, Sprouted Grain Toast, 1/2 Orange
Snack	1 Glass Kombucha, 1/4 Cup Pistachios
Lunch	Beef and Broccoli Leftovers
Snack	Apple, Raw Cheddar Cheese
Dinner	Turkey Mushroom Meatloaf, Side Salad w/Olive Oil and Lemon Juice Dressing

Day 7

Pre-Breakfast	1 Glass Lemon Water/Supplements
Breakfast	Eggs & Sautéed Sweet Potatoes
Snack	Apple, Raw Cheddar Cheese
Lunch	Turkey Mushroom Meatloaf and Side Salad Leftovers
Snack	1 Glass Kombucha, 1/4 Cup Pistachios
Dinner	Quinoa Risotto

WEEK 4 SHOPPING LIST

KOMBUCHA

LEMONS

SPINACH

CELERY

CARROTS

EGGS

CHÈVRE GOAT CHEESE

GOAT or RAW
  CHEDDAR CHEESE

GLUTEN-FREE or
  SPROUTED GRAIN
  BREAD

GREEK or GOAT
  YOGURT (PLAIN)

RAW WHOLE MILK

Apples

Bananas

Oranges

Avocados

Roma Tomatoes

Cucumber

Mushrooms

Green Onions

Onions

Broccoli

Russet Potatoes

Peas

Red Bell Peppers

Green Beans

Mixed Greens for Salad

Sweet Potatoes

Fresh Ginger

Fresh Cilantro

Limes

Chicken Sausage

Chicken Thighs

Salmon

Beef Steaks

Ground Turkey

Low-Sodium Beef Broth

Low-Sodium Chicken Broth

Ketchup

Pistachios

Pine Nuts

Canned Low-Sodium Black
  Beans

Corn Tortillas

RECIPES

RECIPES INTRODUCTION

The following recipes are lunches and dinners you can eat on a regular basis and incorporate easily into a healthy and fast-paced lifestyle. You will notice that many of the recipes include typical meals the average person enjoys such as pizza and burgers, yet these recipes all have unique and healthy substitutions.

Many of the recipes include goat products. Goat products, such as goat cheese and goat's milk, not only taste great, but also provide quality fats and fat-soluble vitamins and minerals. In addition, they are perfect for those with cow dairy allergies who are looking for a comparable substitution.

Make sure to check that all specified ingredients are gluten-free if you are gluten intolerant (such as broths, Worcestershire sauce, etc.)

COCONUT MILK BREAKFAST QUINOA

Serves 2

1 cup quinoa
1 14-oz. can coconut milk
1/8 tsp ground cinnamon

1/8 tsp vanilla extract
1/4 cup toasted coconut
1 cup fresh fruit

METHOD

- ➢ In a medium-sized saucepan, combine quinoa, coconut milk, and cinnamon.
- ➢ As soon as the quinoa reaches a boil, turn the heat to low and cover with a lid for 15 minutes. Halfway through, stir the quinoa a couple of times and place the lid back on.
- ➢ Remove from heat and stir in vanilla.
- ➢ Top with toasted coconut and fruit.

BANANA KALE SMOOTHIE

Serves 1-2

1 banana	2 Tbsp cacao nibs
1 large handful kale	3/4 cup coconut water
1 tsp stevia	1/2 cup ice cubes

METHOD

➤ Blend ingredients together until smooth.

BANANA, ORANGE, AND SPINACH SMOOTHIE

Serves 1-2

1/2 banana

1/2 orange

1 large handful spinach

1/2 cup coconut water

1/2 cup ice cubes

METHOD

➢ Blend ingredients together until smooth.

SUMMER FRUIT & SPINACH SMOOTHIE

Serves 1-2

1 nectarine   1 large handful spinach
1 plum   1/2 cup milk
1/2 banana   1/2 cup ice cubes

METHOD

➤ Blend ingredients together until smooth.

APPLE, GRAPEFRUIT, AND SPINACH SMOOTHIE

Serves 1-2

1/2 apple   1 large handful spinach
1/2 grapefruit   1/2 cup ice cubes
1/2 banana   1/2 cup of milk or OJ

METHOD

➤ Blend ingredients together until smooth.

WHITE PEACH & CARROT SMOOTHIE

Serves 1-2

1 white peach

1 carrot

1/3 cup blueberries

1/3 cup Greek vanilla yogurt

1/2 cup milk

1/2 cup ice cubes

METHOD

➤ Blend ingredients together until smooth.

CREAMY GREEN SMOOTHIE

Serves 1-2

1 banana	1/2 avocado
2 Tbsp peanut butter	3/4 cup milk
1 large handful spinach	1/2 cup ice cubes

METHOD

➤ Blend ingredients together until smooth.

BUTTERNUT SQUASH FRITTATA

Serves 4-6

1/2 of a large butternut squash, peeled and cut into 3/4-inch pieces

1 cup mushrooms, diced

1 large tomato, diced

6 links breakfast sausage, chopped

5 oz. chèvre goat cheese, crumbled

1/2 cup shredded goat or raw milk cheddar

7 eggs, beaten

1/2 tsp basil

1/8 tsp sea salt

1 Tbsp extra virgin olive oil (EVOO)

Fresh cracked pepper

METHOD

➤ Preheat oven to 350 degrees.

➤ In a large skillet, stir fry breakfast sausage and butternut squash with olive oil for approximately 5 minutes or until sausage is slightly browned. Add mushrooms and cook for another minute.

➤ In a medium-sized bowl, mix together eggs, cheddar cheese, salt, pepper, and basil. Combine with cooked butternut squash, sausage, and mushrooms.

➤ Generously coat a medium-sized, oven-safe frying pan with non-stick cooking spray.

➤ Heat pan over medium-high heat and pour in egg mixture. Drop in crumbled goat cheese and spread tomatoes over the top.

➤ Continue to cook for about 3 minutes or until the edges are crispy.

➤ Place the pan into a pre-heated oven and cook for about 20 minutes or until egg is cooked through.

MEXICAN BREAKFAST EGGS

Serves 4

1 15-oz. can black beans, drained

1 15-oz. can diced tomatoes

1 4-oz. can diced green chilies

4-oz. chèvre goat cheese, crumbled

1/2 onion, finely chopped

4-6 eggs

1 Tbsp EVOO

Chili powder

Fresh cracked pepper

Sea salt

METHOD

➤ Preheat oven to broil.

➤ In a large frying pan (with tight fitting lid for later use), sauté onion with olive oil for 2-3 minutes.

➤ Add beans, tomatoes, and green chilies, cover with lid and simmer for 15 minutes.

➤ Stir in goat cheese without letting it melt completely.

➤ Using a spoon, carve out 4-6 indentations to fit each cracked egg.

➤ Crack eggs into pre-formed indentations.

➤ Sprinkle eggs with chili pepper, fresh ground pepper, and salt.

➤ Cover with lid and cook over medium heat for 5 minutes.

➤ Place in oven and broil for another 2-5 minutes depending on desired egg hardness.

TERIYAKI CHICKEN BOWL

Serves 2

6 chicken thighs	3 Tbsp teriyaki sauce
1 tomato, diced	2 cups cooked brown rice
1 avocado, diced	1 cup water
1 Tbsp EVOO	Fresh cracked pepper

METHOD

➤ In a large frying pan (w/ lid), combine the chicken, olive oil, water, 2 Tbsp teriyaki sauce, and pepper. Cook over medium-high heat for 20-25 minutes, covered, flipping 2-4 times.

➤ When chicken is cooked thoroughly, remove from heat and chop into bite-sized pieces.

➤ Layer the chicken, tomato, and avocado over the rice.

➤ Drizzle an extra tablespoon of the teriyaki sauce over the top of the chicken.

QUINOA RISOTTO

Serves 2

1 cup mushrooms, quartered

1/2 cup green beans, sliced
   into 1-inch pieces

1 Tbsp butter

1 Tbsp EVOO

1 cup quinoa

2 cups low-sodium chicken
   broth

METHOD

➢ Heat butter and olive oil in a medium-sized saucepan.

➢ Add quinoa, mushrooms, and green beans and sauté over medium heat for 3-5 minutes, stirring constantly.

➢ Add 1 cup chicken broth and stir regularly until broth is completely absorbed.

➢ Add second cup of chicken broth, stirring regularly until absorbed.

COBB SANDWICH

Serves 1

2-3 slices cooked bacon

1/4 avocado, sliced

2-4 slices turkey/chicken

Handful of fresh spinach

1 medium-sized tomato, sliced

1 hard-boiled egg, sliced

2 slices bread of your choosing

Sliced goat or raw cheddar cheese

METHOD

➢ Layer ingredients to your liking

AVOCADO CHICKEN SALAD

Serves 4

5 chicken thighs

1 avocado

1 tomato

5 strips bacon, cooked

1/2 lime

1/4 cup goat or Greek yogurt

2 Tbsp teriyaki sauce

METHOD

➢ Grill or bake chicken thighs for 15-20 minutes or until cooked thoroughly; brush on teriyaki sauce while cooking.

➢ Chop cooked chicken, avocado, and tomato into approximately 1/4-inch cubes and combine in a medium-sized bowl.

➢ Crush bacon into small pieces; add to other ingredients.

➢ In a small bowl, mix 1/4 cup yogurt and the juice of 1/2 a lime.

➢ Combine yogurt dressing with chicken mixture.

➢ Serve on toasted sandwich bread, over lettuce, or by itself.

TURKEY MEDLEY

Serves 2

3/4 lb. ground turkey
3/4 cup cooked peas
3 handfuls fresh spinach

3 Tbsp of your favorite salad dressing

METHOD

➤ Spray a large frying pan with non-stick spray and cook the ground turkey over medium heat for about 5-7 minutes, regularly stirring and breaking the turkey up into small pieces.

➤ When turkey is fully cooked, add the spinach and cook until wilted.

➤ Remove the pan from heat and add the green peas and dressing, mixing thoroughly.

➤ Serve as is, or over brown rice or quinoa.

GRILLED PORTOBELLO BURGERS

Serves 2

2 medium/large Portobello
  mushrooms
2 Tbsp EVOO
1 Tbsp balsamic vinegar
1/2 cup fresh spinach leaves

1 tomato, thinly sliced
2 oz. cheddar goat cheese,
  sliced (or raw cow's cheese)
1 avocado, sliced
2 gluten-free hamburger buns

METHOD

➤ In a small bowl, combine the olive oil and balsamic vinegar.

➤ On the BBQ or stove top, over medium heat, grill 2 Portobello mushrooms while brushing with the olive oil and balsamic mixture.

➤ Grill evenly on both sides for approximately 8 minutes each.

➤ Assemble your Portobello burger with hamburger buns, avocado, tomato, cheese, and spinach, or any other toppings of your choosing.

QUINOA MEDLEY

Serves 2

2 cups cooked quinoa

1 zucchini

4 hard-boiled eggs, sliced

5 oz. chèvre goat cheese, crumbled

1 avocado sliced into 1/2-inch pieces

METHOD

➤ Cut zucchini in half length-wise, and then into 1/4-inch pieces.

➤ Cook zucchini on stove top in a small frying pan with nonstick spray over medium heat for approximately 5 minutes or until edges are slightly browned.

➤ Combine quinoa, zucchini, hardboiled eggs, goat cheese, and avocado.

SPINACH & GOAT CHEESE CHICKEN BURGERS

Serves 4

1 lb. ground chicken

1/2 cup fresh spinach, chopped

1 tsp EVOO

1/2 cup chèvre goat cheese

1 Tbsp Worcestershire sauce

Fresh cracked pepper

Hamburger buns

METHOD

➢ Sauté spinach with 1 tsp EVOO in pan over medium heat until spinach is wilted.

➢ In a medium-sized bowl, mix spinach, ground chicken, goat cheese, pepper, and Worcestershire sauce.

➢ Hand press mixture into 4-5 burger patties and BBQ (or pan grill) for 3-5 minutes each side over medium heat.

➢ Garnish burger as you like.

CREAMED KALE STUFFED SWEET POTATOES

Serves 2-4

2 large sweet potatoes, baked

4 large handfuls kale, washed and chopped

2 Tbsp butter

1/4 cup Greek yogurt

1/2 cup grated raw cheddar cheese

Salt and pepper for seasoning

METHOD

➤ Preheat oven to broil.

➤ Cut out the top section of the baked sweet potatoes and scoop out insides, leaving 1/4 – 1/2" of potato on all sides.

➤ Sauté kale and butter in a large pan until kale has cooked down, season with salt and pepper.

➤ Remove kale from heat and mix in yogurt and cheese.

➤ Scoop creamed kale into sweet potatoes, top with a sprinkle of grated cheese.

➤ Bake for 10-12 minutes.

SAUSAGE STUFFED PEPPERS

Serves 2

2 green bell peppers

1 1/2 cups cooked brown rice

3/4 cups chicken sausage, chopped

1 cup spinach, chopped

1/2 cup mushrooms, diced

1/2 cup plain goat or Greek yogurt

3 oz. chèvre goat cheese

1/4 cup shredded cheddar goat cheese (or raw cow's cheese)

METHOD

➢ Preheat oven to 375 degrees.

➢ Cut the tops off of the bell peppers and cut in half; remove seeds. Set on a baking sheet sprayed with non-stick spray.

➢ Spray a medium-sized frying pan with non-stick spray and sauté chopped chicken sausage over medium heat until slightly browned.

➢ Add mushrooms to sausage and cook over medium heat for about 2 minutes or until softened.

➢ Add spinach to mushrooms and sausage and cook until wilted.

➢ Transfer the chicken sausage, mushrooms, and spinach to a medium-sized mixing bowl and combine with rice, yogurt, and chèvre goat cheese.

➢ Bake the peppers for 10-15 minutes until softened.

➢ Fill the bell peppers with the sausage mixture, pack tightly.

➢ Sprinkle the shredded cheddar cheese over the top and bake for another 10 minutes.

BALSAMIC GRILLED ARTICHOKES

Serves 2-4

2 large artichokes   2 Tbsp balsamic vinegar
1/4 cup EVOO   1 tsp rosemary
Juice of 1 lemon   Salt and pepper for seasoning

METHOD

➢ Clip off the tips of the artichokes and trim the stem back to about 1 inch.

➢ Steam for 30-40 minutes until just tender.

➢ Let artichokes cool, cut in half, and remove the "choke."

➢ In a small bowl combine olive oil, balsamic vinegar, lemon juice, and rosemary.

➢ Brush the marinade over the artichokes and grill over low/medium heat for 5-10 minutes each side.

➢ Season with salt and pepper.

STUFFED BUTTERNUT SQUASH

Serves 2-4

1 medium-sized butternut
  squash
2 cups mushrooms, chopped
1 large handful fresh spinach,
  chopped
5 oz. chèvre goat cheese

1/4 tsp dried basil
1/8 tsp fresh cracked pepper
Salt and fresh cracked pepper
  for seasoning
2 Tbsp butter

METHOD

➤ Preheat oven to 400 degrees.

➤ Slice butternut squash in half lengthwise and remove seeds.

➤ Place butternut squash cut side up on a baking sheet and place 1 Tbsp butter in each half and season with salt and pepper. Bake for 20 minutes

➤ In a medium-sized frying pan sprayed with non-stick spray, combine mushrooms, spinach, cheese, basil, and pepper, cook over medium heat for 3-5 minutes or until veggies cook down.

➤ After 20 minutes, remove the butternut squash from the oven and stuff the insides with veggie mixture, return to oven and continue to cook for another 15-20 minutes or until squash is easily punctured with a fork.

GRILLED BALSAMIC ZUCCHINI & TOMATOES

Serves 2

2 medium round zucchinis

2 medium tomatoes

8 slices of goat or raw milk cheddar cheese

1/2 cup balsamic vinegar

METHOD

➢ Slice zucchini and tomatoes into 1/2-inch thick sections.

➢ Spray grill with non-stick spray and cook zucchini over medium heat for about 3-5 minutes on each side until just softened.

➢ Grill tomatoes over medium heat for 1-2 minutes on each side.

➢ Layer zucchini and tomatoes with a slice of cheese between each.

➢ Prior to, or while the veggies are on the grill, make the balsamic reduction by heating the balsamic vinegar in a small saucepan over low/medium heat and stirring regularly until the vinegar has reduced down to half its size. Drizzle over stacked zucchini, tomatoes, and cheese.

COLLARD GREENS

Serves 2-4

6-8 collard greens leaves,
  rinsed and roughly chopped

1 small onion, diced

1/2 Tbsp EVOO

3-4 strips of bacon plus
  residual grease

1 medium tomato, chopped

1 Tbsp apple cider vinegar

2 cups chicken broth

METHOD

➤ Fry bacon until crispy (save bacon grease).

➤ In a medium-sized pot, sauté onion until edges are slightly brown.

➤ Add collard greens and bacon grease, sauté for 3-5 minutes.

➤ Add chicken broth and simmer covered over low/medium heat for 25 minutes.

➤ Add tomato, bacon, apple cider vinegar, and another cup of chicken broth and continue to simmer for another 25 minutes, stirring occasionally.

GRILLED SALMON & QUINOA SPINACH SALAD

Serves 2

Two 3-oz. salmon filets

3 cups fresh spinach

1/2 cup cooked quinoa

1/2 large cucumber, sliced in half lengthwise and cut into 1/4-inch pieces

1 avocado, sliced into 1/2-inch pieces

2 Tbsp salad dressing (or lemon juice and EVOO)

1 lemon

2 Tbsp butter

METHOD

➢ Place each salmon filet in a 12-inch long piece of tin foil; add butter and the juice of 1/2 a lemon to each. Close tin foil so each salmon filet is completely wrapped.

➢ Cook the salmon filets over medium heat on the BBQ for 10-12 minutes.

➢ In a medium-sized bowl, mix together the spinach, avocado, quinoa, cucumber, and salad dressing.

➢ Serve salmon over quinoa spinach salad.

YOGURT BROILED HALIBUT

Serves 2

1 lb. halibut filet

3/4 cup grated raw or goat cheddar cheese

3 Tbsp softened butter

1/4 cup Greek yogurt

3 Tbsp lemon juice

3 green onion stalks, finely chopped

1 tsp sriracha

Salt and fresh cracked pepper for seasoning

METHOD

➢ Preheat oven to 425 degrees.

➢ Place halibut in a pre-greased glass baking dish.

➢ Season with salt and pepper.

➢ In a separate bowl combine cheese, butter, yogurt, lemon juice, onion, and sriracha.

➢ In a glass baking dish, evenly coat the fish with yogurt mixture and bake for 12-15 minutes.

LEMON ROSEMARY SALMON

Serves 2

1lb salmon filet

2 lemons, juiced, plus zest

2 tsp rosemary

Salt and fresh cracked pepper for seasoning

2 Tbsp butter

Preheat oven to 450 degrees.

METHOD

> ➤ In a small bowl, combine the zest of two lemons plus the juice.
> ➤ In a glass baking dish, season the salmon with salt and pepper.
> ➤ Pour the lemon juice and zest over the salmon and place thin slices of butter over the salmon.
> ➤ Sprinkle with rosemary and bake for 13-15 minutes or until salmon is cooked through.

ITALIAN BREADED BAKED COD

Serves 2-3

1 lb. cod filet

1/2 cup gluten-free bread crumbs

1 tsp basil

1/2 tsp ground oregano

3/4 cup grated goat or raw cheddar cheese

1 egg, beaten

1/4 cup brown rice flour

1/8 tsp salt

1/2 lemon

METHOD

➢ Preheat oven to 425 degrees.

➢ In a medium-sized bowl mix together the bread crumbs, basil, oregano, cheese, and salt.

➢ Rinse fish and coat with white rice flour.

➢ Dip fish on all sides in the beaten egg.

➢ Coat the fish in the bread crumb mixture and place in a large glass baking dish lightly sprayed with non-stick cooking spray and bake for 10 minutes. Turn the heat up to broil and continue to bake for another 3-5 minutes.

➢ Serve with lemon wedges.

PEANUT BUTTER CHICKEN

Serves 4-6

4 Tbsp butter

2 Tbsp EVOO

3 Tbsp peanut butter

1 tsp red curry paste

1 14-oz. can coconut milk

1 red bell pepper, chopped

2 cups kale, chopped

8 chicken thighs

Salt and pepper

METHOD

➢ In a large frying pan, evenly brown the chicken thighs with 1 Tbsp olive oil and 2 Tbsp butter, season with salt and pepper.

➢ In a small saucepan, whisk together peanut butter and remaining butter over low heat.

➢ Slowly whisk the coconut milk and red curry paste into the peanut butter until thoroughly mixed and smooth.

➢ When chicken is browned on both sides, pour in the peanut butter and coconut milk mixture and simmer covered over medium heat for 20 minutes.

➢ In a separate frying pan, sauté red pepper, kale, and 1 Tbsp olive oil until kale cooks down. Add to chicken mixture for the last 10 minutes of cooking time.

➢ Serve as is or over brown rice or quinoa.

BALSAMIC CHICKEN & TOMATOES

Serves 2

4 chicken thighs

1 cup cherry tomatoes, sliced in half

3/4 cup balsamic vinegar

1 Tbsp EVOO

1 Tbsp butter

1/2 cup low-sodium chicken broth

1/4 tsp basil

Salt and freshly cracked pepper for seasoning

METHOD

> In a medium-sized skillet, melt butter and olive oil over medium/high heat and cook chicken 2 minutes on each side. Season with basil, salt, and pepper.

> Pour chicken broth over the chicken, cover with lid, reduce heat to medium, and continue to simmer for another 20 minutes, flipping chicken halfway through.

> In a small saucepan, heat the balsamic vinegar over low / medium heat and stir regularly until the vinegar has reduced down to half its size.

> When there are about 2 minutes left to cook the chicken, add cherry tomatoes to the skillet.

> Drizzle chicken and tomatoes with balsamic reduction before serving.

FRIED COCONUT CHICKEN

Serves 4

4 chicken breast halves (sliced lengthwise)

1/2 cup organic sulfite-free shredded coconut

1 Tbsp dark brown sugar

1/4 cup gluten-free bread crumbs

1 egg, beaten

5 Tbsp coconut oil

1/4 cup white rice flour

1/4 tsp salt

Salt and fresh cracked pepper for seasoning

METHOD

> In a medium-sized bowl, mix together the coconut, breadcrumbs, sugar, salt, and pepper.

> Rinse chicken and coat in the white rice flour, then dip in the beaten egg, and then coat heavily with the coconut mixture.

> Heat up 3 Tbsp coconut oil in a large frying pan with lid and place chicken in hot oil (careful not to burn yourself). Cover with lid and cook over low heat for 5-7 minutes.

> Flip the chicken and cook for another 3-4 minutes. Add another 2 Tbsp coconut oil to prevent second side of chicken from sticking. Keep covered.

> Serve with your choice of vegetables (shown with sautéed green beans).

QUINOA COCONUT CHICKEN

Serves 2-3

6 chicken legs

1 14.5-oz. can coconut milk

1-2 tsp Thai red curry paste

1 cup low sodium chicken
  broth

1 cup quinoa

1 red bell pepper, diced

1 cup fresh spinach, chopped

1/2 cup mushrooms, sliced

1 onion, diced

1 Tbsp grated fresh ginger

1 Tbsp EVOO

1 Tbsp butter

Salt and fresh cracked pepper
  for seasoning

METHOD

➢ In a large frying pan heat the butter and olive oil and brown chicken on all sides, about 6-8 minutes; season the chicken with salt and pepper while it is cooking.

➢ Remove chicken to a plate, it will continue to cook in step 5.

➢ In the frying pan, sauté the onions until edges are slightly browned.

➢ Add chicken broth, coconut milk, ginger, and red curry paste to the frying pan. Bring to a boil and stir in quinoa.

➢ Add chicken, cover with lid, and cook over med/high heat for 15 minutes.

➢ Give the quinoa and chicken a good stir to scrape off any quinoa that has started to stick to the bottom of the pan. Stir in the bell peppers and mushrooms. Cover and cook on low heat for another 5-7 minutes, gently stirring occasionally.

Turkey Mushroom Meatloaf

Serves 4-6

1 1/2 lbs. ground turkey

1 egg, beaten

2 stalks celery, diced

8 oz. mushrooms, diced

1/4 cup gluten-free bread crumbs

1/2 cup ketchup

2 Tbsp Worcestershire sauce

1/8 tsp fresh cracked pepper

2 green onions, finely chopped

5 oz. chèvre goat cheese, crumbled

Method

> Preheat oven to 350 degrees.

> Mix the celery, mushrooms, green onions, and egg with ground turkey in a large mixing bowl.

> Add gluten-free bread crumbs, ketchup, Worcestershire sauce, ground pepper, and cheese to the turkey mixture.

> Spray a loaf pan with non-stick cooking spray and add the turkey mixture.

> Compact and level the turkey mixture into the loaf pan.

> Bake in the oven at 350° for 1 hour 15 minutes or until cooked through.

CHICKEN FRIED RICE

Serves 4

2 medium chicken sausages,
  sliced into 1/4-inch pieces
1 cup carrots, diced
3/4 cup cooked peas
4 cups cooked rice
2 eggs, beaten

1 Tbsp teriyaki sauce
1/2 Tbsp Worcestershire
  sauce
1/2 red bell pepper, diced
2 Tbsp EVOO
Fresh-cracked pepper to taste

METHOD

➤ Combine carrots, red bell pepper, and 1 Tbsp olive oil; sauté in a large frying pan over medium heat for 5 minutes.

➤ Add chicken sausage and fry until slightly brown.

➤ In a separate frying pan, scramble 2 eggs.

➤ Add rice, 1 Tbsp olive oil, Worcestershire sauce, and teriyaki sauce to the large frying pan and cook over medium heat, stirring frequently until rice reaches desired crispiness.

➤ Stir in the egg and peas and cook over low heat for another minute; add cracked pepper to taste

CILANTRO LIME CHICKEN TACOS

Serves 4

6 chicken thighs
2 Tbsp pine nuts
1 cup washed/dried cilantro
1/4 cup EVOO
2 limes
2 oz. chèvre goat cheese

1 avocado, sliced for toppings
2 Roma tomatoes, sliced for toppings
1 can black beans
Corn tortillas

METHOD

➢ In a food processor, grind up 2 Tbsp pine nuts until they are broken down into a rough paste.

➢ Add the cilantro, olive oil, and the juice of 1 lime into the food processor with the ground-up pine nuts and process until blended smooth.

➢ Add cheese and the juice of the second lime into the food processor and continue to blend until the ingredients are mixed thoroughly.

➢ Refrigerate the cilantro-lime pesto until you are ready to serve the tacos.

➢ Grill, bake, or fry 8 chicken thighs to your liking.

➢ Heat the black beans in a saucepan over low heat until warmed.

➢ After chicken is cooked thoroughly and removed from heat, brush with the cilantro-lime pesto and set aside for 3-5 minutes.

➢ After the pesto has set on the chicken, slice chicken into thin slices and build tacos with corn tortillas, cilantro-lime chicken, avocado, tomatoes, and black beans.

➢ Add additional cilantro-lime pesto to your tacos as you like

ENCHILADAS W/ TANGY AVOCADO CREAM SAUCE

Serves 4

2 cups cooked chicken, cubed or shredded

4 brown rice tortillas

1 14-oz. can low-sodium refried beans

1 14-oz. can red enchilada sauce

2 cups grated goat cheddar or raw cheddar cheese

4 large handfuls fresh spinach

1 cup mushrooms, diced

1/2 Tbsp EVOO

1 large avocado

1/2 cup Greek yogurt

2 limes

METHOD

➢ Preheat oven to 350 degrees.

➢ In a medium-sized frying pan, heat the olive oil and sauté mushrooms until just soft. Add the spinach and cook down.

➢ Warm up the brown rice tortillas in the microwave until they are easy to roll without breaking (suggestion: try layering each tortilla with a damp paper towel to keep moist; microwave about 20 seconds).

➢ On each tortilla, evenly layer the refried beans, chicken, cheese, mushrooms, spinach, and a couple of spoonfuls of enchilada sauce.

➢ One-by-one, roll up the tortillas and place next to each other in an 8 x 8" glass baking dish lightly sprayed with non-stick cooking spray.

➢ Pour the remainder of the enchilada sauce over the top and down the sides.

➢ Sprinkle the remaining cheese over the top and bake for 20 minutes.

➢ In a food processor, combine 1 large avocado, Greek yogurt, and the juice of 2 limes; use as a topping.

BEEF & BROCCOLI

Serves 2

1 lb. grass-fed beefsteaks cut into 1/4-inch strips

1/2 onion, diced

2 cups broccoli florets

1 cup mushrooms, quartered

1 cup low-sodium beef broth

1/3 cup teriyaki sauce

1/2 Tbsp organic brown sugar

1 Tbsp Worcestershire sauce

1/2 Tbsp fresh ginger, peeled and shredded

1 Tbsp EVOO

METHOD

➢ In a small bowl, mix together teriyaki sauce, brown sugar, Worcestershire sauce, ginger. Set aside.

➢ In a large non-stick frying pan, sauté onion with olive oil until softened and edges are browned.

➢ Add the steak and the sauce mixture to the onion and continue to cook over medium heat for 5-7 minutes.

➢ At the same time, in a separate medium-sized frying pan, simmer broccoli and mushrooms with beef broth covered with a lid over medium heat for 3-4 minutes.

➢ Strain the vegetables from the beef broth and add to the beef. Continue to simmer together for another minute.

EASY BBQ PORK RIBS

Serves 2-4

2 small racks of pork ribs   3 Tbsp Worcestershire sauce

METHOD

➢ BBQ ribs over low heat for 2 to 2 1/2 hrs.
➢ In the last 15 minutes, brush on Worcestershire sauce.

VEGETABLE & WILD RICE SOUP

Serves 4

6 chicken thighs

1 qt. low-sodium chicken broth

1 cup water

7 oz. canned coconut milk (optional)

1/8 tsp pepper

1/4 tsp salt

1/4 tsp dried basil

1/2 cup wild rice

1/2 cup brown rice

1/2 onion, diced

1 1/2 cups carrots, sliced

1 cup mushrooms, quartered

1 cup celery, sliced

METHOD

➢ In a large pot, season chicken with salt, pepper, and basil.

➢ Add rice, chicken broth, water, and onion to the pot and cook over med/high heat covered for 30 minutes.

➢ Add celery, carrots, and mushrooms, and continue to cook over low heat with lid on for another 20 minutes.

➢ Stir occasionally to break up the chicken into bite-sized pieces.

➢ After 20 minutes, stir in the coconut milk and let simmer for another 5 minutes.

BACON LENTIL SOUP

Serves 4-6

2 cups lentils	4 slices cooked bacon, chopped
4 cups low-sodium chicken broth	1 cup mushrooms, sliced
4 cups water	1/4 tsp dried oregano
1 cup carrots, sliced	1/4 tsp dried basil
3 celery stalks, sliced	14-oz. can diced tomatoes
1/2 onion, diced	1 Tbsp butter

METHOD

➢ In a large pot, melt butter and sauté onions until slightly browned.

➢ Add lentils, chicken broth, and water, and simmer, covered, over low/medium heat for 60 minutes.

➢ Add carrots, celery, mushrooms, diced tomatoes, basil, and oregano and simmer for another 30 minutes.

➢ Remove from heat and stir in bacon; let sit 5-10 minutes before serving.

CHEESE & BROCCOLI SOUP

Serves 3-4

2 Tbsp butter

1 cup grated carrots

1/2 onion, finely diced

2 celery stalks, chopped

2 small russet potatoes, cut into 1-inch pieces

5 1/2 cups low sodium chicken broth

1 1/2 Tbsp brown rice flour

2 1/2 cups broccoli, chopped

2 cups grated goat or raw cheddar cheese

Fresh cracked pepper to taste

METHOD

> In a large pot, sauté carrots, celery, and onion with butter for about 5 minutes or until the veggies are slightly tender.

> Add the potatoes and 5 cups chicken broth to the pot. Cover and cook over medium heat for about 15 minutes or until the potatoes are slightly tender.

> Mix the remaining 1/2 cup chicken broth and flour separately in a small bowl and add to the soup; stir well.

> Add the broccoli and continue to cook covered over medium heat for another 10 minutes, stirring often.

> Add the cheese and fresh cracked pepper; stir well.

> Let sit 5 minutes uncovered before serving.

NO CARB LASAGNA

Serves 4-6

1 1/2lbs ground chicken

1 28-oz can crushed tomatoes

1 14-oz. can diced tomatoes

1 red bell pepper, diced

1 yellow bell pepper, diced

1 tsp dried basil

1/8 tsp ground oregano

4-6 handfuls fresh spinach

2 cups sliced mushrooms

1/2 Tbsp EVOO

4 oz. chèvre goat cheese

2 cups grated goat or raw cheddar cheese

METHOD

➤ Pre-heat oven to 375 degrees.

➤ Spray a large pot/frying pan with non-stick spray and cook ground chicken until just cooked.

➤ In a separate frying pan, sauté bell peppers with olive oil until slightly blackened on the edges.

➤ Add bell peppers, crushed tomatoes, diced tomatoes, basil, and oregano to the ground chicken.

➤ Simmer with lid on low for 20 minutes.

➤ Add 2 oz. goat cheese and stir well.

➤ Spray a 9 x 18" glass baking dish with non-stick spray.

➤ Divide the tomato chicken sauce into 3 parts and layer as follows: tomato chicken sauce, spinach, grated cheese, more tomato chicken sauce, mushrooms, spinach, grated cheese, and top off with another layer of tomato chicken sauce, grated cheese, and remaining chèvre goat cheese.

➤ Bake for 20 minutes, turning the broiler on for the last 3-5 minutes.

SPINACH ARTICHOKE MAC N' CHEESE

Serves 2-3

1 quart low-sodium chicken broth

4 cups water

12 oz. gluten-free penne pasta

1 14-oz. can artichoke hearts (cut into 1/2-inch pieces)

8 oz. frozen, chopped spinach

2 1/2 Tbsp butter

2 Tbsp brown rice flour

2 cups milk

1 1/4 cup grated goat cheddar

Fresh cracked pepper to taste

METHOD

- ➤ Preheat oven to 400 degrees.
- ➤ Bring chicken broth and water to a boil; cook pasta until al dente and drain.
- ➤ In a small saucepan melt butter, whisk in flour, and slowly whisk in milk a 1/2 cup at a time over low heat.
- ➤ When sauce has thickened, add 1 cup cheese and stir until melted.
- ➤ In a large pot, combine pasta, cheese sauce, spinach, and artichokes.
- ➤ Evenly coat an 8 x 8" glass baking dish with non-stick cooking spray, evenly spread out pasta mixture, top with remaining cheese.
- ➤ Bake for 15 minutes and turn on broiler for last 3-5 minutes.

BASIL PESTO PASTA W/ BBQ CHICKEN

Serves 4

6 chicken thighs

2 cups fresh basil, rinsed and dried

3 Tbsp pine nuts or raw almonds

3/4 cup EVOO

4 oz. chèvre goat cheese

1/8 tsp fresh cracked pepper

1/4 cup teriyaki sauce

1 Tbsp Worcestershire sauce

Brown rice pasta to serve 4

1 Tbsp butter

METHOD

➤ In a food processor, grind 3 Tbsp nuts until finely ground.

➤ Add basil and 1/4 cup of olive oil to food processor and blend until smooth.

➤ Add cheese, another 1/2 cup of olive oil, and pepper to food processor and blend.

➤ Set pesto aside in a separate container and refrigerate until pasta and chicken are ready (you will have extra pesto that you can freeze for future use).

➤ Combine teriyaki sauce with Worcestershire sauce and brush onto chicken while cooking on BBQ, about 20 minutes over medium heat.

➤ Cook enough pasta for 4, drain, rinse, toss w/ butter and pesto to your liking.

➤ Serve with chicken.

CAULIFLOWER MAC N' CHEESE

Serves 4

2 heads cauliflower, broken into bite sized florets

1 1/2 cups milk

2 cups grated goat or raw cheddar cheese

3 Tbsp butter

3 Tbsp brown rice flour

1/2 cup gluten-free bread crumbs

1 tsp dried basil

1/8 tsp dried oregano

1/8 tsp salt

1/8 tsp fresh ground pepper

METHOD

➤ Preheat oven to 375 degrees.

➤ Steam cauliflower for 5-7 minutes until slightly tender.

➤ In a small bowl, mix together bread crumbs, basil, oregano, salt, and pepper.

➤ In a medium saucepan, melt butter over low/medium heat and whisk in flour. Gradually whisk in milk a 1/2 cup at a time letting the mixture thicken each time.

➤ Whisk cheese into milk over low heat until completely melted. Remove from heat.

➤ Mix together the cauliflower and cheese sauce.

➤ Spray an 8 x 8" glass baking dish with non-stick spray and spoon in half of the cauliflower mixture.

➤ Sprinkle half the bread crumb mixture over the cauliflower, layer with the rest of the cauliflower and top with remaining bread crumbs.

➤ Bake in oven for 12-15 minutes, turning broiler on for last 2 minutes.

Spaghetti Squash w/ Turkey Meatballs

Serves 4

1 lb. ground turkey

1 1/2 cups mushrooms, chopped into 1/4-inch pieces

2 green onions, finely chopped

1 cup fresh spinach, chopped

1 egg, beaten

2 Tbsp Worcestershire sauce

5 oz. chèvre goat cheese

Fresh cracked pepper to taste

1/8 tsp ground oregano

1 spaghetti squash

1 jar marinara sauce (or follow recipe for tomato sauce listed in the roasted pepper and eggplant lasagna recipe)

Non-stick cooking spray

Method

➢ Preheat oven to 350 degrees.

➢ Cut spaghetti squash in half, lengthwise, scoop out seeds, place cut side down in a glass baking dish. Fill with 1/2 inches of water.

➢ Bake at 350 degrees for 45-50 minutes until softened.

➢ In a large bowl, stir together ground turkey, mushrooms, green onions, spinach, egg, Worcestershire sauce, pepper, goat cheese, and oregano.

➢ Spray a baking sheet w/non-stick cooking spray.

➢ Form the turkey mixture into 2-inch round balls, pack tightly, spread evenly on the cookie sheet, and bake for 30-40 minutes. Note: It is okay to cook spaghetti squash and meatballs in oven at same time on different racks.

➢ When the spaghetti squash is cooked, move to a plate and scrape the spaghetti squash out into thin strands with a fork.

➢ Serve squash and meatballs with your choice of sauce.

CAULIFLOWER PIZZA

Serves 4

2 heads of cauliflower

2 cups grated goat cheese

3 eggs

1 Tbsp EVOO

1/4 tsp basil

1/8 tsp ground oregano

1/2 cup marinara sauce

METHOD

➢ Cut cauliflower away from stem and into 1-2 inch pieces.

➢ Steam cauliflower for approximately 20 minutes or until cooked through.

➢ In a large bowl, use a mixer to mash up the cauliflower.

➢ Add the 3 eggs, 1 cup cheese, basil, and oregano. Mix well.

➢ Spray a cooking sheet with non-stick spray and then use a brush to evenly coat the cooking sheet with olive oil.

➢ Pour the cauliflower mixture onto the baking sheet and use the brush to evenly spread to the edges.

➢ Bake at 400 degrees for 25-30 minutes or until edges are crispy and top is slightly browned.

➢ Top with marinara sauce and cheese. Continue to bake for another 5-10 minutes or until cheese is melted and slightly browned.

ROASTED PEPPER & EGGPLANT LASAGNA

Serves 4

1 lb. ground chicken

1 large or two small
  eggplant(s)

1/4 tsp ground oregano

1/4 tsp basil

1/8 tsp fresh cracked pepper

1/2 cup goat or Greek yogurt

10 oz. chèvre goat cheese,
  crumbled

6 (15 oz.) cans diced
  tomatoes

1 red pepper

1 green pepper

1 tsp Celtic sea salt

METHOD

➤ Preheat oven to 400°.

➤ Simmer 6 cans diced tomatoes in large saucepan over medium heat, stirring occasionally, for 45 minutes.

➤ Cut off the tops of the red and green bell peppers, remove seeds, and slice in half lengthwise. Place the peppers cut side down on a baking sheet sprayed with non-stick spray.

➤ Place the peppers in the oven and bake for 30 minutes or until the skins are turning black and bubbling away from the meat of the red pepper.

➤ Remove from oven and let cool until you can safely remove the skins.

➤ Dice peppers into 1/4-inch pieces.

➤ Spray a separate frying pan with non-stick spray and cook the ground chicken over medium heat until browned.

➤ Peel the eggplant(s) and slice into 1/8-inch pieces lengthwise. Sprinkle with salt and set aside.

➤ After the tomatoes have been simmering for 45 minutes, use a masher to break up the large chunks.

➤ Add the cooked ground chicken, oregano, basil, pepper, yogurt, and diced peppers to the tomatoes and remove from heat.

➤ Spread a thin layer of the tomato sauce in the bottom of a 10 x 15" baking dish. Layer half of the sliced eggplant on top of the tomato sauce, then spread tomato sauce over the eggplant and 5 oz. of the goat cheese over the tomato sauce.

➤ Repeat layering of eggplant, sauce, and goat cheese until all ingredients are gone. Bake for 40 minutes; broil for the last 5 minutes.

➤ Remove from oven and let sit for 10 minutes before serving.

TURMERIC CHICKEN

Serves 2-3

6 chicken legs

Zest and juice of 1 lemon

1 cup Greek yogurt

1 tsp turmeric

Pinch of chili powder

1 Tbsp EVOO

1 Tbsp rosemary

METHOD

> ➤ Preheat oven to 375 degrees.
> ➤ In a small bowl combine lemon, yogurt, turmeric, chili powder, and olive oil.
> ➤ Spray a glass baking dish with non-stick spray, place chicken inside, and coat evenly with yogurt mixture.
> ➤ Sprinkle rosemary on top of chicken.
> ➤ Cook for 40 minutes, flipping the chicken halfway through.

ROASTED PEPPER SNACK BITES

Serves 4-6

1 red bell pepper, sliced into
1-inch pieces

1 yellow bell pepper, sliced
into 1-inch pieces

1 large avocado, sliced into
3/4-inch pieces

1/2 cup grated goat or raw
cheddar cheese

METHOD

- ➤ Preheat oven to 400 degrees.
- ➤ Lightly coat a baking sheet with non-stick cooking spray and evenly lay out the cut bell peppers; bake for 10-12 minutes until just getting soft.
- ➤ Place a piece of avocado on each pepper and top with cheese.
- ➤ Turn oven to broil and place peppers back in oven for 3-5 minutes; watch carefully that they don't burn.

BACON AVOCADO DEVILED EGGS

Serves 4-8

4 eggs, hardboiled, cooled,
and peeled

1/2 avocado

3 strips bacon, cooked and
crumbled into 1/4-inch
pieces

2 Tbsp Greek yogurt

2 tsp white vinegar

1 Tbsp yellow mustard

Salt and fresh cracked pepper

METHOD

➢ Slice eggs in half lengthwise and remove yolks into a
medium sized bowl.

➢ With a fork or electric mixer, combine the egg yolks,
avocado, two-thirds of the bacon crumbles, yogurt, vinegar,
mustard, and a generous amount of salt and pepper until
smooth.

➢ Scoop the mixture into the egg whites and top with
remaining bacon crumbles.

EASY CUCUMBER SALAD

Serves 2

1 medium cucumber, sliced lengthwise and into 1/4-inch slices

Juice of 1 lemon

1 Tbsp EVOO

1 Tbsp parsley, finely chopped

1/4 tsp apple cider vinegar

Salt and fresh cracked pepper to taste

METHOD

➢ In a small bowl, combine lemon juice, olive oil, parsley, and apple cider vinegar.

➢ Pour lemon juice mixture over sliced cucumber and season with salt and pepper.

VEGETARIAN LETTUCE WRAPS

Serves 4

8 oz. tempeh

1/2 cup carrots, shredded

2 cups mushrooms, finely chopped

2 Tbsp EVOO

1 head of butter or iceberg lettuce

2 Tbsp teriyaki sauce

1/2 Tbsp brown sugar

1/2 Tbsp Worcestershire sauce

1 Tbsp ketchup

1/8 tsp garlic powder

METHOD

➤ Cut tempeh into 1/4-inch to 1/2-inch pieces.

➤ Combine tempeh, carrots, mushrooms, and olive oil in a medium-sized skillet and stir-fry over medium heat for 5 minutes.

➤ Combine teriyaki sauce, brown sugar, Worcestershire sauce, ketchup, and garlic powder in a small bowl and add to tempeh mixture. Cook for another 5 minutes.

➤ Wash individual lettuce leaves and serve as lettuce wraps with tempeh mixture.

BROCCOLI & CARROT SLAW

Serves 4

2 1/2 cups shredded broccoli

1/2 cup shredded carrots

1/2 cup Greek yogurt

1 Tbsp honey

2 Tbsp lemon juice

1 Tbsp balsamic vinegar

Salt and pepper to taste

METHOD

➤ In a large bowl, combine broccoli and carrots.

➤ In a small bowl, combine yogurt, honey, lemon juice, balsamic vinegar, salt, and pepper.

➤ Toss the broccoli and carrots with the Greek yogurt mixture, cover, and let sit in fridge for 3-4 hours before serving.

ROASTED ALMOND BUTTER

Makes 3 cups

2 cups raw almonds

8 cups water

2 Tbsp coconut oil (as needed)

1 tsp sea salt

1 tsp stevia

METHOD

➤ In a large bowl soak almonds and water for at least 12 hours.

➤ Dry almonds with a towel and bake in oven for 10-12 minutes at 350 degrees.

➤ Pour the almonds into a food processor and blend on high for 15 minutes (if you feel the mixture is too dry after 15 minutes, add coconut oil until you reach your desired consistency).

➤ Mix in sea salt and stevia for added flavor.

➤ Store in the refrigerator.

CINNAMON APPLE CHIPS

Makes 2 cups

3 apples   1 tsp cinnamon
1/4 cup coconut sugar   Juice of 1/2 a lemon

METHOD

➤ Preheat oven to 225 degrees.

➤ Core and thinly slice apples.

➤ Place apples in a zip lock bag and toss with lemon juice.

➤ In a small bowl, combine cinnamon and sugar.

➤ Coat apples with cinnamon and sugar mixture and place on baking sheets lined with parchment paper.

➤ Bake for 1 hour, turn apples to other side, and cook for another hour. (If you want the apples very crispy, bake for 1hr 15 minutes each side)

➤ Leave apples in the oven, turn heat off and let sit until the oven cools.

PERFECT COCONUT OIL POPCORN

Serves 1-2

1/3 cup popcorn kernels   Salt and butter to taste
3 Tbsp coconut oil

METHOD

> ➢ In a medium-sized saucepan, heat the coconut oil over low to medium heat.
> ➢ Add 2-4 popcorn kernels and cover with lid.
> ➢ When the popcorn kernels have popped, remove from heat and add remaining 1/3 cup popcorn kernels.
> ➢ Cover with lid and let sit for 30 full seconds.
> ➢ Place pot back on heat and the remaining kernels will start popping.
> ➢ Gently shake the pan back and forth until there are a few seconds between pops then remove from heat. As the kernels are popping, keep the lid slightly ajar to let some steam out.
> ➢ Pour the popcorn into a bowl, season with salt and melted butter to your liking.

BAKED ZUCCHINI STICKS

Serves 4-6

3 zucchini, each sliced into 8 sections

1 cup gluten-free bread crumbs

1/2 cup shredded goat cheddar cheese

1 Tbsp dried basil

1/2 Tbsp ground oregano

2 eggs, beaten

1/2 cup white rice flour

Fresh cracked pepper

1/2 tsp sea salt

METHOD

➢ Preheat oven to 400 degrees.

➢ In a medium-sized bowl, combine the bread crumbs, cheese, basil, and oregano.

➢ Line three bowls up next to each other, the first containing the flour, the second the eggs, and the third the bread crumb mixture.

➢ Coat each zucchini stick first in the flour, then egg, then the bread crumb mixture and place onto a baking sheet sprayed with non-stick spray.

➢ Cook in oven for 30 minutes, turning every 10 minutes to bake each side evenly.

SPINACH ARTICHOKE DIP

Serves 8-10

2 cups frozen chopped
   spinach
1 14-oz. can artichokes, diced
1 red bell pepper, diced
5 oz. chèvre goat cheese

1 cup goat or Greek yogurt
Juice of 1 lemon
1/8 tsp pepper
1/4 tsp salt

METHOD

➤ Preheat oven to 400 degrees.

➤ In a large bowl, mix together all ingredients.

➤ Spray an 8 x 8" glass baking dish with non-stick cooking spray.

➤ Evenly spread mixture into glass baking dish with a spoon and bake for 25 minutes until it is bubbling at the edges.

PEANUT BUTTER PROTEIN BARS

Makes 12-16 snack bars

1 egg, beaten	1 1/2 cups gluten-free oats
2 Tbsp softened butter	1/2 cup peanut butter
1 cup vanilla goat yogurt	1/3 cup chocolate chips

METHOD

- ➢ Preheat oven to 350 degrees.
- ➢ In a medium sized bowl beat the butter until creamy with an electric mixer.
- ➢ Add the egg, vanilla yogurt, and peanut butter; mix until smooth.
- ➢ With a wooden spoon, mix in the oats and chocolate chips
- ➢ Spray an 8 x 8" glass dish with non-stick cooking spray and spread the protein bar mixture into the pan evenly.
- ➢ Bake for 25 minutes.

COCONUT OIL CHOCOLATE

Serves 4-6

3/4 cup coconut oil
3/4 cup cacao powder
3/4 cup coconut sugar
1 tsp vanilla extract

1 Tbsp butter
1/4 cup sulfite-free coconut flakes

METHOD

➤ Toast the coconut in a small saucepan over medium heat.
➤ Grease the bottom and sides of an 8 x 8" glass baking dish with butter.
➤ Set the toasted coconut aside and add the coconut oil, cacao powder, and sugar to the small saucepan.
➤ Over low heat, whisk for about 2-4 minutes until ingredients are mixed thoroughly.
➤ Remove from heat and add the vanilla and toasted coconut.
➤ Pour the chocolate into the glass baking dish and put in freezer for 20 minutes.
➤ Remove from freezer and sprinkle with sea salt. Put back in freezer until it is completely solid then break into pieces

BANANA ZUCCHINI MUFFINS

Makes 2 dozen muffins

3 eggs

1 cup raw sugar

1 cup softened butter

1 1/2 cups brown rice flour

1 1/2 cups white rice flour

1/2 tsp salt

1 tsp baking soda

1/4 tsp baking powder

1 1/4 tsp vanilla

2 cups grated zucchini

2 very ripe bananas

METHOD

➤ Preheat oven to 350 degrees.

➤ In a large mixing bowl combine the flours, salt, baking soda, baking powder and mix with a spatula or wooden spoon.

➤ In another large mixing bowl mash the bananas with an electric mixer, then add the eggs, butter, sugar, and vanilla and mix until smooth.

➤ Using the electric mixer, add half the wet mixture with the dry, mix all the way together then add the remaining wet mixture and mix until smooth.

➤ Add the grated zucchini and stir with a wooden spoon or spatula.

➤ Spray 2 medium-sized muffin tins that will hold a dozen muffins each with non-stick spray and evenly distribute mixture.

➤ Bake for 30-40 minutes.

YOGURT BLUEBERRY MUFFINS

Makes 1 dozen muffins

1 cup brown rice flour

1 1/4 cups white rice flour

2 Tbsp white rice flour

1/4 cup coconut sugar

1 1/2 tablespoons baking
  powder

1 tsp salt

2 eggs

1 cup goat or Greek yogurt

1/2 cup butter

1/3 cup milk

3 Tbsp lemon juice

1 1/2 tablespoons lemon zest

1 1/2 cups fresh blueberries,
  rinsed and drained

Glaze:

  1 tsp lemon juice

  1/4 cup confectioners'
    sugar, sifted

METHOD

> Preheat oven to 400 degrees.

> In a large bowl, combine 1 cup brown rice flour, 1 1/4 cup white rice flour, coconut sugar, baking powder, and salt. Set aside.

> In a medium bowl, whisk together eggs, yogurt, butter, milk, 3 Tbsp lemon juice, and zest.

> Gently mix together the wet and dry ingredients until just combined.

> In a small bowl coat the blueberries in 2 Tbsp white rice flour, fold into batter.

> Lightly spray a 12-cup muffin tin with non-stick cooking spray and fill each cup with approximately 1/3 of the batter. Bake for 25-30 minutes.

> To make the glaze, whisk together 1 tsp lemon juice and 1/4 cup confectioners' sugar. Make sure to sift the sugar or your glaze will be lumpy.

> Brush the lemon glaze over the cooled muffins.

PUMPKIN SNACK BARS

Makes 12-16 snack bars

3 Tbsp butter, softened

1/4 cup coconut sugar

1/2 cup applesauce

2 eggs

1 14-oz. can pumpkin puree

1 tsp vanilla

1 cup brown rice flour

1 cup white rice flour

1 tsp cinnamon

1/4 tsp nutmeg

1/4 tsp ginger

1 tsp baking soda

1/2 cup chocolate chips

METHOD

> Preheat oven to 350 degrees.
> In a medium bowl, combine flours, cinnamon, nutmeg, ginger, and baking soda.
> In a large bowl, combine the butter, sugar, applesauce, eggs, pumpkin, and vanilla with an electric mixer.
> Slowly mix the dry ingredients into the wet ingredients until mixed well.
> Stir in the chocolate chips.
> Spray an 8 x 8" glass baking dish with non-stick cooking spray and evenly spread in the pumpkin mixture.
> Bake for 35-40 minutes.

HEALTHY CARROT CAKE

Serves 12

1 cup applesauce

1/4 cup butter, softened

1 cup coconut sugar

3 eggs

1 tsp vanilla

1 cup brown rice flour

1 cup white rice flour

1 tsp baking soda

1 1/2 tsp baking powder

1/2 tsp salt

1 tsp cinnamon

2 cups grated carrots

1 cup grated coconut

1 cup crushed pineapple

Glaze:

   1 Tbsp milk

   1/4 cup powdered sugar, sifted

   1 cup shaved coconut, toasted

METHOD

- Preheat oven to 350 degrees.
- In a large bowl, mix applesauce, butter, coconut sugar, vanilla, and eggs.
- In a medium bowl, combine white and brown rice flour, baking soda, baking powder, salt, and cinnamon.
- Gradually mix the dry ingredients into the wet ingredients.
- Stir in the carrots, coconut, and pineapple.
- Pour into a greased 9 x 13" baking pan and bake for 35-40 minutes or until a toothpick comes out clean.
- To make the glaze, combine the milk and powdered sugar, mix well with a whisk.
- Brush the glaze over the top of the cake
- Top with toasted coconut.

METHODOLOGY OF EXERSCRIBE

The Exerscribe training model involves taking the body through phases.

Poor motor skills and poor posture degrade your ability to move properly. The Movement Efficiency Phase addresses this issue by integrating more bipedal (upright) and rotational movement patterns, which helps mobilize and stabilize the critical joints of the body (i.e., ankles, knees, hips, and spine). This phase is also characterized by slower tempos in order to crystallize better motor skills and brain-muscle connections.

After a strong foundation has been established, we take you through the Force Optimization Phase, where an eclectic variety of forces are applied to the musculoskeletal system. The goal of this phase is to maximize the progressive overload of forces displaced on the body for optimal strength and muscular development.

The Mechanical Synergy Phase is characterized by faster tempos and velocities, with an emphasis on hand-eye and foot-eye coordination. The speed-, agility-, and quickness-specific drills assigned in this phase are designed to bring out your inner athlete – taking your fitness to new heights.

The nucleus of the entire system is optimizing stress tolerance and well-being. Not just mental and emotional stressors, but also the physical stressors from unstable joints and chemical stressors from poor nutrition. Our Conscious Variation™ provides your nervous system adequate stimulation and strategic workout variety to prevent plateaus. The body adapts to exercise programs every four to six weeks, which is why we progress your workout every month.

Our NanoProgression™ technology customizes your workout experience and tailors it to your individual needs and preferences.

The Tempos and Durations specified for each exercise in our workouts maximize the results you gain from each rep.

The Corrective function digs deep to treat root causes to problems by addressing your potential pain areas with relevant corrective exercises on the spot. After completing your assigned corrective exercise and resetting the nervous system's pain-threat response, we take you back to your original workout so you don't skip a beat.

Life Lines gamify your experience as a utility by giving you ten opportunities in each workout to get an extra minute of rest when you really need it.

By focusing on behavioral-based metrics like Fitness Capacity % (how much of the assigned workout you completed), we expect your outcome-based metrics (i.e., weight and body fat) to be achieved inherently.

No Gimmicks. No Quick Fixes. Just Results. **Exerscribe.com**

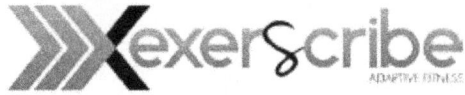

SAY 'HELLO' TO YOUR NEW WORKOUT PARTNER

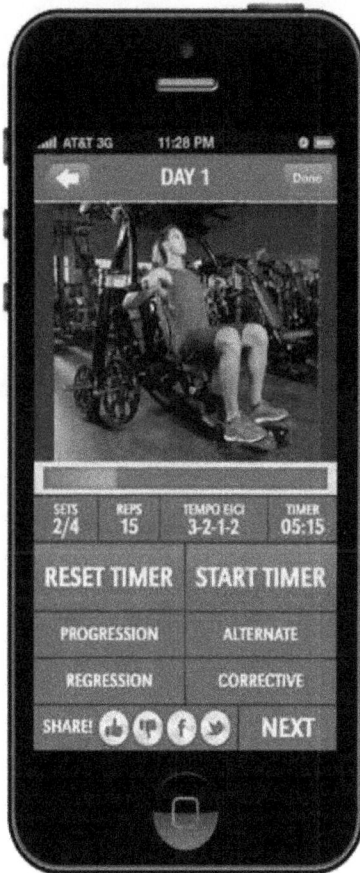

ACKNOWLEDGEMENTS

Kelley and I thank you for reading *Eat Fat, Get Fit* and sincerely hope the philosophies contained here have had a positive impact on your life the way they have on ours.

Please take a moment to share your thoughts with us about the book by leaving a review on Amazon. This will not only help us in future writings, but also help get this book into the hands of others.

Thank you again for reading *Eat Fat, Get Fit.*

JOIN US!

This book was brought to you by the creators of Exerscribe, a company dedicated to the biohacking movement.

What is biohacking? Hacking is about creating the shortest path to success through optimization. Biohacking is about reaching new limits, maximizing your true potential, and becoming "superhuman."

No longer can we solely rely on the information from doctors or the FDA. It's our responsibility to gain the highest level of truth for our health and wellness by getting the best information possible – information that has no hidden agendas.

Join our biohacking revolution and subscribe to our newsletter at **exerscribe.com** today.

No spam or scams, you have our word.

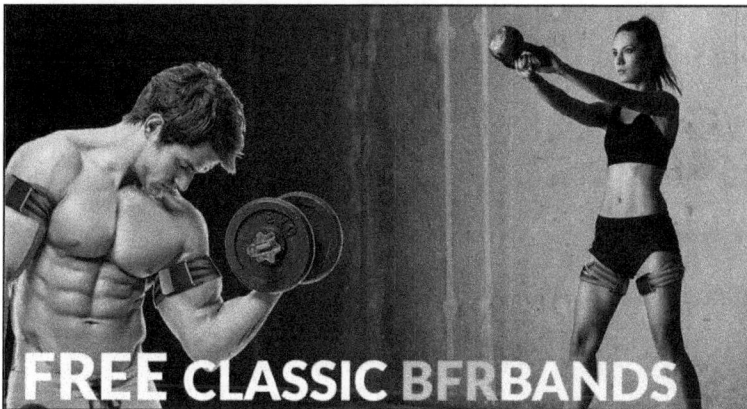

ABOUT THE AUTHORS

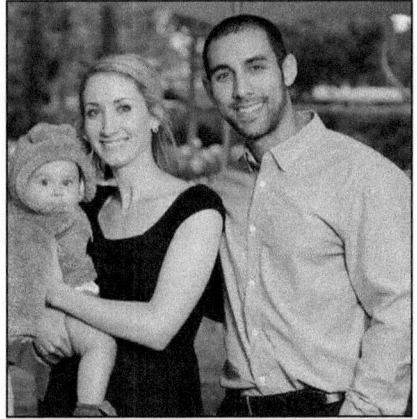

Kusha Karvandi is an entrepreneur and fitness enthusiast and has worked as a professional trainer and health club manager in the San Diego area for six years. As the founder of Exerscribe, Kusha has made it his business to teach the truth about fitness and living a healthy lifestyle across the globe. This book brings together many of the nutritional insights and guidelines developed by and practiced by Kusha and his wife, Kelley.

Kelley Karvandi has a background in design and project management, yet has a keen interest in nutrition as medicine. Over the years, through trial and error, Kelley developed the collection of healthy recipes that are the cornerstone of this book.

Together, the two share a passion for fitness, nutrition, healthy living, and their son Preston.

GET BOOK DISCOUNTS AND DEALS

Get discounts and special deals on our bestselling books at

www.tckpublishing.com/bookdeals

REFERENCES

NOTES

[1] Taubes, Gary. *WHY We GET FAT AND WHAT TO DO ABOUT IT.* NEW YORK: Knopf, 2010

[2] Ross, Julia. The Mood Cure: The 4-Step Program to Take Charge of Your Emotions – Today. New York: Penguin, 2003.

[3] IBID.

[4] IBID.

[5] IBID.

[6] Braly, James, and Ron Hoggan. Dangerous Grains: The Devastating Truth About Wheat and Gluten and How to Restore Your Health. New York: Avery, 2002.

[7] IBID.

[8] Enig, Mary, and Sally Fallon. *EAT FAT, LOSE FAT: THE HEALTHY ALTERNATIVE TO TRANS FATS.* New York: Hudson Street Press, 2005

[9] Cowan, Thomas, Sally Fallon, and Jaimen McMillan. *THE FOUR-FOLD PATH TO HEALING: WORKING WITH THE LAWS OF NUTRITION, THERAPEUTICS, MOVEMENT AND MEDITATION IN THE ART OF MEDICINE.* WHITE PLAINS, MD: New Trends Publishing, 2012

[10] IBID.

[11] ROSS, *THE MOOD CURE.*

[12] Cowan, Fallon, and McMillan, *The Four-Fold Path.*

[13] Price, Weston A. "The Weston A. Price Foundation." *Weston A. Price Foundation*. Accessed April 6, 2017, www.westonaprice.org.

[14] Price, Weston. NUTRITION AND PHYSICAL DEGENERATION (8TH ED.). LEMON GROVE, CA: Price-Pottenger Nutrition Foundation, 2009.

[15] IBID.

[16] "COMMUNITY SUPPORTED AGRICULTURE." LOCAL HARVEST. ACCESSED APRIL 6, 2017, WWW.LOCALHARVEST.ORG/CSA .

[17] "ECONOMIC JUSTICE FOR FAMILY-SCALE FARMING." CORNUCOPIA INSTITUTE. ACCESSED APRIL 6, 2017, http://www.cornucopia.org.

[18] Warinner, Christina. (2013, February 12). "Debunking the Paleo Diet: Christina Warinner at TEDxOU." YouTube video, 22:19. Posted by TEDx Talks, February 12, 2013. http://www.youtube.com/watch?v=BMOjVYgYaG8

[19] Brownstein, David. *Salt Your Way to Health* (2nd ed.). West Bloomfield, MI: Medical Alternatives Press, 200).

[20] Ding, Sarah. "Celtic Sea Salt: Health Benefits." *Juicing for Health*. March 21, 2017. http://juicing-for-health.com/sea-salt-health-benefits.html

[21] Berardi, John. "Precision Nutrition." *Precision Nutrition*. Accessed April 6, 2017, http://www.precisionnutrition.com

[22] D'Adamo, Peter, and Catherine Whitney. Eat Right 4 Your Type: The Individualized Diet Solution to Staying Healthy, Living Longer & Achieving Your Ideal Weight. New York: Berkley, 1996.

[23] BERARDI, "PRECISION NUTRITION."

[24] Asprey, Dave. "Introducing Bulletproof Intermittent Fasting: How to Lose Fat, Build Muscle, Stay Focused & Feel Great." *Bulletproof*. October 26, 2012. Retrieved December 1, 2013, from www.bulletproofexec.com/bulletproof-fasting.

[25] Berardi, "Precision Nutrition."